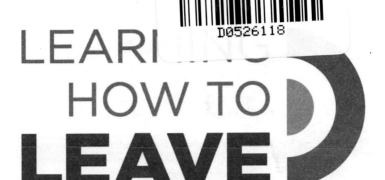

LEARNING
HOW TO
LEAVE

A Practical Guide to Stepping Away from Toxic Narcissistic Relationships

MICHAEL PADRAIG ACTON

B.Ed., M.Ed. (Psych.) Hons., M.A. C.Psych., P.D. C.Psych., BPSsS., BACP (Accred), MICF

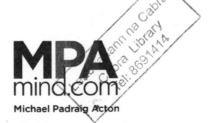

MPA
mind.com
Michael Padraig Acton

Published by Life Logic Publishing 2021

Text © Life Logic Publishing 2021
Illustrations © KS Turner 2021
Cover Design © Helen Braid 2021

A CIP catalogue for this book is available from the British Library.

Paperback ISBN 978-1-8383527-0-7

Typeset in Garamond Classic 11.25/14 by Blaze Typesetting

Printed in Great Britain by Clays Ltd, Elcograf S.p.A.

When a narcissist accuses you of something,
it's truly a confession. . .

ACKNOWLEDGEMENTS

I would like to start by thanking my clinical supervisors who have really made a difference to myself and my patients over the years.

First, Ruth Baker BACP Snr Accrd. Ruth has been an amazing mentor and guide with fantastic skills to navigate me through my clinical cases with care, insight and reflection. She beautifully combines this with supporting my personal wellbeing, enabling me to go all out.

I also give thanks to Gary Taylor and Brenda Roberts from the Royal Sussex Hospital Psychology Dept., St Peters Place, Brighton, East Sussex and Morley Street Children's Clinic. I learnt so much and your support was second to none.

Then, there are my scholastic mentors. From Stirling, I thank all members of the education faculty that gave me the opportunity of cementing my first career path. I fondly recall Angela Rogers from Dundee University.

"You just missed a first by three points Michael," was Angela's response as I stood in a telephone box having called in to see if I had failed my Master's degree in Psychology and Education. Silence prevailed.

She was so helpful, supportive, encouraging and knowledgeable about how to get the best out of me. I truly could not have juggled and managed everything without her firm and nurturing support. I again learned so much.

Moving on to Mick Burton from Sussex University. Bless Mick's soul. He departed soon after I completed my Master's degree in Counselling Psychology. He opened a door to the psychoanalytic world and the field of applied psychodynamic therapy. He was a gentleman and a true scholar.

Mic Cooper was an amazing supervisor for my controversial research at Sussex and Brighton universities. He showed me how to mould and develop a hypothesis and how to best interview participants to generate themes and ideas. This has helped me immeasurably during my career. I am so pleased he went on to become a professor and a major contributor to the field of counselling psychology.

I also want to mention Malcolm Cross from London City University. I felt that there was a huge gap in my knowledge and ability to work with people throughout all aspects of their struggles. It was Malcolm's encouragement as my Director of Studies that sent me along the path of systemic therapy, which involved relationship and family work. He opened up a whole new world for me and also helped me to become a much more effective therapist. I never work with people in isolation; Milanian Systemic Principles have guided me well to work with people in their context.

And lastly, there is John Waite from the University of Western England. John taught me so much about poor supervision practice and how to learn from his examples and be an 'effective' supervisor myself. In the group supervision he mentored, John highlighted how the need for confidentiality is paramount to enable people to safeguard students, patients and faculty staff. I supervise carefully and effectively due to the lessons I learned.

FOREWORD

Michael has brilliantly sewn this book on codependency and narcissism together. The dance that occurs between the codependent and narcissist is couched with such elegance that all who read this book will feel that they are dancing right along with them. The couple whose story we follow through the course of the book depict the true nature of the narcissist and codependent relationship. It's eye-opening to be able to witness this relationship from a distance, as a reader and an observer.

From the moment Michael introduces these characters to us, we're able to consciously feel the stark differences between the two of them. We are able to get a sense of the two personalities. . . and that entices us to look deeper and read on. How Michael delicately draws them into conversation and then into showing their true motivations for therapy is masterful. As we read along, we cannot help but feel as if we're sitting alongside Michael, looking upon his patients, from his perspective.

The dialogue that permeates through this book creates the ideal place to learn from.

Michael has more than three decades of clinical and counselling experience and that is clearly seen, as we are drawn into his clinical examples with such ease. This is a brilliantly constructed book on a topic that so many authors are unable to articulate for their readers.

I am a paediatrician with 18 years of experience in applied knowledge and clinical experience as a physician, community paediatrician and researcher.

Throughout my years of clinical practice I have worked

with a multitude of codependent and narcissistic relationships. Looking for a book on this topic was difficult to find, let alone one that I could learn from.

After reading *Learning How To Leave* my eyes have been opened again to looking at how I approach and then dance with my patient relationships. I am able to offer new avenues for my patients and families that will create healing and understanding. Michael has created this book for all to read and learn from.

I highly recommend this book and I will be offering it to the families I serve and especially my peers in the medical world.

Barry Scott Lowy
MD Paediatrician

AUTHOR'S NOTE

Many books dealing with Narcissistic Personality Disorder (NPD) focus solely on the narcissist and the pathological traits behind their behaviour; less attention is paid to the other side of the coin: the codependent.

To understand the basic pattern of the narcissist-codependent relationship, think of the two individuals as dancers at an evening party. The narcissist is the perfect lead on the dance floor: confident, self-assured and decisive. They engage with everyone, asking each in turn to dance, yet none of the dance partners quite match up. Perhaps they misread the narcissist's movements and step on their toes, or are too rigid to just enjoy being swept away in the moment. Finally, the narcissist approaches the humble codependent who has been watching all along—as if mesmerised—from the shadows. A moment later, the narcissist is asking the codependent to dance.

The codependent, amazed at their luck, accepts the invitation and, within minutes, the two are gracefully sweeping around the room.

The acquiescent codependent watches their partner's every step with the care and attention they have grown up learning to provide. The pair adapt and move perfectly together and the dance seems effortless and a joy to watch. The narcissist laps up the attention from their partner and those who are watching in awe. The codependent, carried away by the drama and romance of it all, believes that they have met the partner of their dreams and waits for the day when the narcissist looks back at them, eyes brimming with mutual respect and love—but that moment never comes.

They try ever harder to prove their worth as a dance partner, yet the narcissist barely recognises the effort, wrapped up as they are with how they appear to others around them. As bitterness grows and self-esteem crumbles, the codependent looks across the dance floor for options but sees no one looking back; fear paralyses them. They realise they will never find anyone as eligible as the narcissist and so must choose between being alone in the shadows of life or continuing in a dance that no longer holds any enjoyment for them bar the glimmers of hope that keep them there (*'Who would ever love me?'*). The narcissist has now completely taken control, reaffirming the codependent's childhood fears of being unlovable.

The key to the codependent is their self-destructive belief that they are responsible for their significant other's happiness or misery. They lack the ability at this point to separate out and see the whole 'damned' picture.

This is the moment when they become trapped—unless they can find a path to healing the wounds that are behind their maladaptive behaviour. NPD and codependency transcend all genders and sexualities.

There is hope for peace and happiness but if you are reading this book for a codependent you know (or for yourself) they will already be in the grip of distorted thinking.

It is my sincere hope that this book, compiled through years of scholastic and evidence-based therapeutic practice, enables the suffering codependent to realise their predicament and to take their first steps upon that healing road. In recognition that readers of this book may not be seasoned academics, I have deliberately kept my language plain and concise, and let the case examples do much of the talking. This focus on readability, accessibility and linguistic economy is a seam that runs through this *Power Of You* series, of which this is the first book. My aim is to open up taboo topics and bust myths surrounding real-life problems that face the people I've been working with over the past 30 years, from toxic relationships and domestic abuse to parenting guilt and grief. The *Power Of You* series aims to reach people in their homes, wherever they are, so I can share my experience and offer support via these pages to everyone who needs it. This has always been my calling. And the *Power Of You* books are written from the heart for every single person who needs them.

Thank you for reading,

Michael Padraig Acton

PROLOGUE

I still cannot believe that I have been working for more than 30 years in the therapy world, most of which I have spent studying and training in one form or another. My thirst for knowledge stimulates me and helps me to deliver my very best to my clients and via my writing. I have loved every moment of my work and I am enjoying the opportunity to write books and share all that I have been taught during my practice.

Throughout this time working in mental health with families, couples and young people, I do not think there is a setting I haven't worked in. My experience has ranged from hospitals, inpatient wards, pain clinics and prisons (during my clinical psychology training days) to drug dependency units, HIV/AIDS clinics, child protection units, family centres, children's clinics, dioceses and, of course, private practice.

I have also helped lawyers represent people in mediation and litigation; I don't think there is one type of court out there I have not experienced either.

Supporting people with relationship breakdowns, helping children see better futures, nailing a perpetrator or unhooking people from criminal actions and abuse is my life's work.

I wonder, at times, how I did it all, especially having no support from parents and being a single parent for most of my daughter's upbringing.

During our toughest years, I worked four jobs, juggled childcare and never thought anything of it; I had the strongest and ever-present need to give my daughter a better start in life than me. I did my best by her, for sure, and that is all any parent can expect; to be good enough.

I was going to be a Catholic priest up until the age of 14, when my childhood experiences started to challenge my image of the church, my school, the nuns, brothers and priests. All of a sudden, nothing made sense. A massive shift occurred. I stopped serving at church.

It was a big step: the church and its cloth had been my teachers and source of safety in my childhood world of chaos, danger and abuse.

My Aunt Violet (the kindest soul who encouraged my reading and love of crossword puzzles) taught me that I could learn and do anything that I found in a book. I was a strange kid. I had 10 encyclopaedias that I would read, opening pages randomly to satisfy my fascination for knowledge.

It was like having a curtain cracked open that showed me the wonders and possibilities outside of my own—then—dark and tiny world. This is how I self-soothed, how I survived. I imagined great comfort in faraway lands and science. I spent hours searching online. Google is my miracle!

At 16, while living in Eire (Ireland), I struggled for many months to survive meningitis. I then returned to England and my UK family home and somehow, at that moment, found the strength to leave (run away). I lived in a friend's car for six weeks; I never went back 'there'. I was free. I did not know what from back then, I just knew it tied me up in knots and I had to leave. It was toxic.

A month into sleeping rough and my worldly possessions consisting only of a blanket, floppy pillow and a few plastic bags with clothes in, I awoke one morning to the freezing cold; the type of cold only found in England at three-thirty in the morning inside a rickety old car. My nose and my ears were hurting.

All of a sudden, I had an awakening, a true and sudden awareness. It was like I was completely enveloped in wonder and light—everything tingled. The scriptures in church could never have put words to what happened in that moment. I realised, for the first time in my life, that I was *free*. I was in complete control of *everything*. I could do and be anything I wanted. My mind was freed up. I knew I was done with the past—done with surviving in a trapped and dark place.

Later that very same day, I found a bedsit (tiny studio apartment) with a shared toilet, sink and kitchen. Devi Breeze, a midwife and landlady in Gravesend, Kent had given me my first step up in life. Devi took a chance on me, this 17-year-old kid, by renting out this tiny space. It was mine, my special kingdom, a safe place in which I could read, better myself and plan, which is exactly what I did.

After much thought about how I was going to earn reasonable money and have a good life with a good standing, I decided my best option was to become a teacher. It seemed to be a noble profession. I could also do a teaching Diploma and fast-track into work.

I read The Guardian newspaper's education section every week at Gravesend Library. I wondered at all the international jobs that were advertised around the world for teachers, realising that education would be my ticket. I was a waiter and barman to make ends meet, a great choice for observing, listening intently to and taking note of the well-heeled customers and their stories. I recreated myself; learned how to be.

After experiencing teaching for a while, I realised that I was on the wrong side of the desk and that education just wasn't stimulating for me. I felt like a puppet, pumping out the same thing, day in and day out. I wasn't a naturally gifted teacher.

While working at a college in Sydney, Australia, I chose student pastoral care as part of my job's extracurricular role. I had no training; I just had to be available to students who might be in trouble or have attendance issues. I loved it. I just found it so rewarding and interesting. I read extensively about various pathways into doing this full time.

I had naturally been the listening ear for many of my friends. People would tell me their stories and confide in me so I already felt I had a gift in this area. It fitted, in fact, it felt like a comfy, old pair of slippers. I found it so rewarding, interesting and challenging.

I looked for universities and planned to do a conversion course to become a graduate member of the British Psychological Society and to then go through clinical training.

I chose Dundee University and Dundee Royal Infirmary hospital. Within four months, I had been accepted, relocated and found a place to live. It felt so good to be back on track. I did a pre-course counselling certificate in Edinburgh. My insight into and comprehension of mental health and life's challenges began.

We had little money and I was surviving on pure faith and hope that things would work out. I have since apologised to my daughter, as going back into full time education and working multiple jobs put a strain on our lives. I regularly went to the Middle East on small contracts in order to earn the money for fees and living. My daughter knew no different and recounts many of the places she visited with me as "interesting" or "special".

Fast forward to narcissism and codependency. Even though I have had extensive training in the Diagnostic and Statistical Manual of Mental Disorders (DSM) and the International Statistical Classification of Diseases and Related Health Problems (or International Classification of Diseases for short - ICD10), I never connected or clicked that myriad areas of this training mirrored my childhood and adult relationships.

Even my training and daily work with couples and families showed me the warnings, terrors and absolute destruction NPDs cause people and how codependents were thwarted. For decades I kept dating and living with NPDs. I repeated this pattern of toxic relationships for years and years. It was familiar and, I thought, normal.

I was living a parallel universe. Helping people by day and living my own relationship horrors by night. Of course, it took me the longest time to understand in my gut that it was *my* codependency that was getting me hooked every time! My own codependency fuelled my belief that no one could love the real me, that I was lucky to have 'love' and, worst of all, that bad things happened to me because I was intrinsically bad.

I over-compensated for my own childhood by giving my all to others, rescuing them until there was nothing left for me. What drove me to write this book was the hope that my being candid, scholarly and genuine may help a lightbulb go on for someone out there who is also caught in this. I was soon to realise that I had escaped NPDs when I was 17 but had continued to recreate that unhealthy and destructive—but familiar and oddly comfortable—relationship. Over and over, like a cruel drug.

The pattern became clear one day while I was working

with a couple. I saw how word for word, action for action they were mirroring my life with my then partner. So, I did something about it. Oh boy. That withdrawal was the most painful and the most liberating. As soon as I made the cut I saw everything so clearly and what was more potent, people close to me affirmed it was the right move and had wondered if I ever had a clue that this was happening to me or that it was painful for them to watch. Some NPDs cover their tracks very well but most end up letting their shield down just enough for the horrors to be seen.

So, what I am sharing with you in this book not only comes from my formal training, spiritual awakening and the immense knowledge that I have gathered from my amazing and brave patients over the years. It also comes from my own experiences of being a codependent in relationships with narcissists.

I am now happily married and peaceful in my life but it took work, relapse, wondering and challenging my core beliefs and coping mechanisms. And then it also took every morsel of my being to get unhooked; to stop being a caring and kind feeding source for an NPD. Quite a counterintuitive place for me to be, but my kindness and 'unconditional love' ran dry. I had been used and abused to the point of 'done'.

It was difficult for me to not complete the final year of my professional doctorate. From the young age of 21 and the birth of my daughter, I had to work to eat.

I could never have taken the time and definitely did not have the money to do a PhD, even though I was offered several places over the years to do so. This would have been my Narnia.

Five years ago, I consulted a life coach. I felt doing a PhD and working in a faculty would be a great way to give back all that I have learnt over the years. I have a successful global private practice and now work as a consultant with people on a part-time basis. So I could do it. At last.

However, the outcome of those coaching sessions was for me to give back to people who aren't able to afford therapy, cannot access therapy for other reasons, or just don't want to. I feel, again in my gut, that this is a third cathartic awakening in my life. The writing of these books is my way of giving and of adding to the field of psychology, psychiatry and psychotherapy. My contributions are from very real cases and very brave people who decided to change their lives and the lives of those they care for.

I am blessed and fortunate. I left school with very few qualifications, found my voice at 17 and with determination and listening to my soul, I am pretty happy with the way I 'made' things turn out.

These books are my PhD and I give my grateful, heartfelt thanks to those people that entrusted me with their personal struggles! I am truly humbled.

I dedicate every word of this to all of you who have inspired and helped me in my life journey and those still to come. Thank you sincerely. . .

"Being a codependent is like having high blood pressure.
It is a silent killer."
-Michael Padraig Acton-

CONTENTS

More games and gaslighting
The colour of hope
Inside a narcissist's mind: a true case of dangerous NPD development

PART II: DIFFERENT PERSPECTIVES: NARCISSISM AND CODEPENDENCY OUTSIDE OF THERAPY

Chapter 7. Four unique lenses
No accounting for narcissists by Loretta Fabricant
Courting disaster by Sarah Zabel
Personal agency by Jim Davis
Mother knows best by Barry Scott Lowy

Chapter 8. Managing codependency in the workplace
Recognising and dealing with codependent traits
The effect of narcissists in the workplace
The NPD and codependency dance at work

Chapter 9. Narcissism & codependency in business partnerships
Beware the career narcissist by Marty Davis
The importance of personal attributes for team success
Narcissist at the helm: a case study
Learning lessons: the mark of the career narcissist
Resolving a bad business arrangement

Chapter 10. Avoiding domestic violence: tracking, tracing and stopping the narcissist
What does NPD abuse look like?
Where are we with domestic violence?

An important note on teenage relationship abuse
Joining the dots
The elusive narcissist: a warning from Oliver Twist

Chapter 11. Joining the dots of domestic violence and NPD: a meeting of minds by Susan Weitzman and Michael Padraig Acton

Breaking the mould
"The veil of silence"
A key to healing
Getting the message out

PART III: UNHOOKING & RECOVERING FROM A NARCISSIST

Chapter 12. Breaking the dynamic: how do I quit you?

Codependency, addiction and self-loathing
Addiction and the DSM-5
Spotting the patterns
The role of motivation

Chapter 13. The unhooking process

Six stages of change
Stepping away is the only path to healing
What next if you realise you need help?

Chapter 14. A better way to be: creating new boundaries to move forward

Love, unity and compassion
You live the life you accept for yourself

SUCCESS MANTRA

Ralph Waldo Emerson made such an immediate impact on me at an early age that I have used his words as my success mantra for as long as I can remember:

To laugh often and much
to win the respect of intelligent people
and affection of children;
to earn the appreciation of honest critics
and endure the betrayal of false friends;
to appreciate beauty,
to find the best in others;
to leave the world a bit better,
whether by a healthy child, a garden patch
or redeemed social condition;
to know even one life has breathed easier
because you have lived.
This is to have succeeded.

-Ralph Waldo Emerson-

PART I

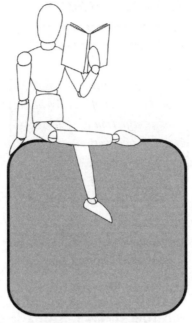

UNDERSTANDING NARCISSISM & CODEPENDENCY

CHAPTER 1

DEFINING NARCISSISM

*"Sometimes we need to throw that stone and call the judgment
and just see things and people for what they are!"*
-Michael Padraig Acton-

Introduction

Many people will find themselves in a less than happy
relationship, at times. It is all part of being in a relationship.
Many of us tough out the difficult times with the great times
and the boring times. But when a relationship becomes
unhealthy, sad, stuck, upsetting, demoralising, suffocating,
even dangerous, and you are still in it; this generally means
that you are a codependent living with a narcissist.

An independent person who has healthy boundaries would
tell a toxic partner to go, take the high road and not look back.
The toxic person would have no further use for an independent
person as their ego and imaginary world would starve. If you
are reading this and recognise you are in this unmistakably

stuck place, grieving for love and normality, read on. I'll help you make sense of this situation and your role in it.

I am a narcissist. . . and so are you at times.

When I have a cold, for example, I think only about my own needs and can be overly demanding on those I care about.

But I don't have Narcissistic Personality Disorder (NPD).

Everybody can be bipolar at times too. When shook by grief, for example, people will often plunge to the depths of depression on some days before rebounding and feeling in control, even wonderful, on others.

We don't all have bipolar disorder though.

Since my first book on narcissism, we have seen an explosion of interest in the subject. It seems that any person who ever lies, cheats, steals, ignores our feelings or blames us for a problem, is now labelled a narcissist.

Who does this serve?

Every diagnosed disorder can be 'managed' with drugs and unfortunately this is now the norm.

Doctors are mostly diagnosing patients with these disorders after seeing them for only 10 minutes. This behaviour is certainly a boost for the drugs companies. All you need to do is look at the news and TV programmes to see how we are bombarded with quick-fix drugs promising us a miracle cure.

Unfortunately, a large majority of codependents who approach me for help are already comatose from being prescribed a cocktail of anti-anxiety and anti-depressant drugs, primarily by their General Practitioner (GP) or Internist, for years!

All prescription drugs for anxiety and depression require (it's on the Patient Information Leaflet) regular management by the prescriber, and are only to be prescribed as an adjunct to psychotherapy. This very rarely happens and it should be a crime. It keeps people quiet and is the best, cost-effective way to reduce patient waiting times. Desperately sad, but true!

The media also benefit, demonising the powerful and successful as hedonistic, abusive, egotistical narcissists because it makes for juicy headlines and stories.

But it certainly doesn't help those people trapped in the deadly dance of the narcissist-codependent dynamic, the people I see in my clinics and you, reading this book.

Some might argue that shining a light on narcissism and codependency is a good thing—and it could be. But when the terms are thrown about like confetti, the real victims get confused. And since codependents are hard-wired and have been trained to support the narcissists in their denial, if the fuzzy, shifting pattern doesn't fit exactly—well, they couldn't possibly be a narcissist, could they?

The reason I chose NPD and its victims as the subject of this first book in the *Power of You* series of accessible self-help books is because of the abhorrent, bloody, evil, lethal actions I've witnessed (there are just no words that can describe the horrors I have seen in my practice helping victims and, at times, working with NPDs as part of a family). There is no cure for an NPD. I repeat, there is no cure to NPD. They just change tack, make us believe there is some remorse or apology and, bang, they are back with another self-centred, self-serving game plan. I hope my voice, through this book, will be cathartic for all those souls that have been/are suffering from the unimaginable grip of their evil.

In this book, I place even more focus on the hidden,

suffering codependent. Codependents are critical to the understanding of narcissism because an NPD can only exist as part of a relationship. They hop from host to host each time they deplete every ounce of what they wish to take. Remember, they are only done with you when *they* believe they are. They will stalk you and try to damage you in any way they can.

If something is wrong in your relationship—if you are hurting and you can't understand why—this book is written for you.

I hope to break through to you, as you need to start thinking seriously about your position and recognise that there are some basic practical steps you can—and must—take to start planning your escape. Now!

It is going to take steady work and clear navigation. We need to consider both our need for safety and our emotions.

Only caring for our safety kills our heart, but only caring for what's in our heart is dangerous.

Every year, I find myself grabbing metaphorically drowning people by the hair and metaphorically slapping them round the face and pulling them to safety.

If this book can do the same for those millions of people I can never hope to see personally via my work, this will be my success.

I am fascinated by the accounts I hear from other professionals working in fields as diverse as law, finance, medicine and business. My work often has me as part of a team involving lawyers, forensic accountants, medical doctors, teachers, social workers and child protection units.

These people recognise the existence of NPD and codependency in their professions but their experiences vary from mine, due to the nature of their working relationships with their narcissistic or codependent clients. I also recognise that their angle, ideas, opinions and frameworks are very different to mine due to those working relationships, as well as their laws, their policies and their outcome focus. I felt it would therefore be super helpful if their voices were included in this book.

Narcissism and codependency not only transcend all genders and sexualities, as mentioned before, but also all types of relationship and all of life's contexts.

I am so very grateful that a collection of these esteemed professionals, when asked, came forward willingly and most passionately to enrich these pages. There are helpful accounts from a business lawyer, life coach, medical doctor, judge, corporate employee and forensic accountant.

The central structure of the book is built around a central case study—one which typifies the narcissist-codependent relationship (although please remember that a narcissistic relationship can be between any two people, not just spouses and partners, it could be a friendship, a family member, a working relationship etc).

Also be mindful that toxic relationships can be insidious and an NPD-codependent relationship can creep up and develop without us knowing it. Clear case examples are used to show specifics, although it is not always as clear cut as is sometimes stated or suggested.

The couple featured is not one couple. It is a collection of situations combined to create a core story, which is typical and tragically very real—and one that repeats itself in similar ways across very different situations. The case study material is presented to be read as one narrative.

Be mindful, NPD, like all personality disorders, is a controversial area within psychology and psychiatry and no experts have all the answers or necessarily agree. I hope this develops more questions for our profession that will eventually inform more effective practice.

NPDs provide domestic violence, mental health issues and sometimes death to their victims.

My patients have included prosecuting attorneys, celebrities, TV show hosts, magazine writers, big names from the pop psych field, drug companies, rock bands, the film world, therapists, psychiatrists, prisoners, gentry and public figures of all shapes and sizes. Beware, no one is safe if they have kindness and unhealthy boundaries. Due to embarrassment and fear, codependents are left mostly to suffer in silence, denying themselves the voice and the understanding that could set them free.

As with all of my writing, this is a real book written from real people's experiences, including my own. I am grateful for everyone's feedback as this has helped form this first book in the *Power of You* series.

I hope you find benefit in reading this most comprehensive, practical, easy-to-follow guide to freedom from narcissism.

Narcissism and codependency: a therapist's insight

To me, my rooms often feel like cavernous wells, where people pour in their pitchers of ideas, stories and viewpoints along with their many assorted feelings, thoughts and aspirations. Everyone in life has their own stories and, clearly, no one completely escapes the ruggedness of their time on this planet.

From desperation to enlightenment, our journeys take us down many pathways.

I often have people present to me who identify narcissistic traits in their partner, parent or child and, at times, even worry that they see these qualities in themselves. Truth is, we all have narcissistic traits; it's part of being human and also one of our most necessary defences against harm.

Think about it: when we catch a miserable cold, study for an exam, prepare for a special meal or even work on the garden after a hard winter, we must focus and give our all to that project—at that time. Nothing exists for us apart from our own needs and wants (unless of course an emergency should arise). 'Our' world is all that matters and we need the rest of the world to understand that 'we', and what's immediately at hand for 'us', come first and everyone else needs to agree on its importance and support us. When we are in depression or illness, we focus on ourselves, our issues and our needs; we often burn out friends and people close to us because we drone on and on about our loss, our difficulties, our struggles and our blame.

It is normal and healthy to be egocentric at times—all about 'me, me, me'—but if we don't have NPD we get that this cannot go on and sooner or later, we restore a balance between our own needs and those of others. However, someone with NPD will feel that this attention is, and always will be, their given right and underneath their mask, will feel no emotion towards the plight of another.

Nevertheless, they are capable of sending out all the right signals to those outside their familial context and have a well-rehearsed ability to charm, say the right things and to generally be the 'belle of the ball.'

When I publish articles on certain aspects of narcissism, what generally follows is a swift spike in referrals/enquiries from people who are really suffering from the impact of such unhealthy relationships.

These people, in immense pain, will identify with much of what I write about narcissism. Now, this need not be about their partner: it can also be about a significant other such as their own child, grandchild or parent, or a close friend. Narcissism, and narcissistic traits, know no boundaries and narcissists may impact any and all who are close to them. I can work with narcissists on their problematic traits to a degree: NPD is an attitude that has developed from early childhood and I can help narcissists in their attempts to manage it, in order to improve life for them and their significant others. But, in my experience, narcissism is not something we, as therapists, can eradicate in our therapy rooms.

To be in a significant relationship with someone with NPD is to be in a very confined and extremely lonely place.

As a codependent, you need to know that it is fear and need that are keeping you safe in this familiar dance or dynamic—but fear and need will not keep you happy, content or emotionally safe in the long-run.

Even as I'm writing this, I can feel the deep, stomach-churning despair, the chest-tightening panic and the dark loneliness that accompanies the hopeless nature of being around this danger.

Narcissism in Psychiatry
Let's look at some definitions. NPD is one of 10 specified Personality Disorders in the DSM-5 main manual.

According to the manual:

Personality disorders are associated with ways of thinking and feeling about oneself and others that significantly and adversely affect how an individual functions in many aspects of life. (1)

This definition is important! A disorder of any type can only be diagnosed if there is a negative impact on that person's life (which includes their relationships). It is not enough to display narcissistic traits—there has to be dysfunction, risk or actual harm.

The DSM divides Personality Disorders into clusters.

These can help to refine diagnosis but are of most interest to the drugs companies looking to match a label with a type of medication. The labels switch about now and then with new disorders added and separated out while others are removed or merged together. If you find yourself getting confused between a narcissist and someone with a borderline personality, don't get lost in the fog. If your relationship is suffering, seek out a therapist experienced in working systemically with couples and families.

Therapists are focused on improving relationships and reducing risk—not behavioural management through meds.

Narcissism is as old as the hills and will always be with us, despite how its definition may change in the DSM.

For now, NPD is classed as one of four 'Cluster B' mental disorders, the so-called, 'dramatic, emotional, erratic cluster,' where it sits alongside Antisocial Personality Disorder (ASPD), Histrionic Personality Disorder (HPD) and Borderline Personality Disorder (BPD).

As with all personality disorders in the DSM-5, NPD is characterised by both an impairment of personality and unhealthy traits. Specifically, narcissists:

- Draw their identity and self-esteem from others. They use others to hold up an inflated or deflated opinion of themselves. This self-appraisal can fluctuate between the two poles with emotions swinging up and down in response.
- Set goals based on their (often unrecognised) need for approval.
- Their standards are either impossibly high or, conversely, appallingly low (since they feel entitled to special treatment so feel no need to make any effort).

In relationships, narcissists:

- Have little empathy with the needs and feelings of others.
- Take notice of others' reactions only if it directly affects them.
- Have limited awareness of the effects of their actions on others.
- Are only superficially involved, using intimacy as a way to regulate self-esteem.

The pathological (harmful) traits of NPD are:

- Antagonism, due to an exaggerated self-importance and an overt or hidden sense of entitlement (grandiosity).

This can cross over into violence and 'narcissistic rage' if their self-esteem is wounded.
- Attention-seeking, with a need to be admired by others.

As I mentioned in the introduction, everyone is narcissistic to a degree, although popular books from the last decade (e.g. *Generation Me* and *The Narcissism Epidemic*) point the finger particularly at those born in the 1980s and 1990s.

However, any psychiatric diagnosis of NPD requires symptoms that go beyond what is expected from the person's stage of development, their social background and the temporary effects of any legal or illegal drugs. NPD always shows itself within a relationship and always results in harm.

What does narcissism and codependency really look like on the front line?

Find some space, sit down, relax, and let's look at our first case study.

It was early Spring, with just an edge of bitter cold in the air commingled with the freshness of the sun, which streaked across Earl's Court Square in London, as I walked to my rooms, familiar and comforting to me after my having practised there for almost two decades.

I picked up my regular coffee to welcoming smiles from the familiar people at the local coffee house; I habitually weighted down my coffee with nutmeg, cinnamon and three Sweet 'N Lows.

The mixed spice aroma was warming; it was a perfect moment to start preparing for my day.

I crossed the street, opened the iron gate and descended the cold, hard stairs to the big blue entrance door. My first new intake of the day was clearly following close behind for, as soon as I set down my coffee and began to get out my files and various accoutrements for the day, the door buzzer went.

Now, patients are asked to be no more than 10 minutes early. This is to help protect the identity of those patients finishing their sessions and also to help minimise interruptions. But this intake was 35 minutes early!

Some people travel significant distances at times, even using long-haul flights, so I usually suggest that they use my local coffee shop to gather themselves before arriving; but today a man and a much younger woman were already standing there and shuffling slightly, so I welcomed them in, asked them to take a seat and said that I would be with them at 10.00—their allotted time.

I returned to my room and continued my ritual of setting up for the day.

I have used the same, now straggly, clipboard for many years. It displays the emblem of one of my first universities and still serves me well as a hard surface on which to write my session notes.

Every day is new; my work is never dull. I never know what to expect from the individuals, couples and families I work with, particularly with new intakes. I walked into reception and into an atmosphere that could have been cut with a knife but my new couple both rose, with beaming smiles and outstretched hands, and introduced themselves.

They were both well-groomed and smartly dressed, they

had clearly made an effort to make a positive impression. They were also very forward and charming.

This gushing level of charming can, at times, signal warning bells for me. It feels fake. It feels over the top. It could be compensation for nervousness but largely this 'well-rehearsed, leaning forward, shaking of hand, big smile, everything's perfect' approach usually symbolises to me a massive cover-up for something that is difficult, abhorrent and worth hiding. Most people are anxious and, if anything, a little humble coming to see me (it's part of the stigma of seeing a shrink, let's be honest!).

So, when people are overconfident, approaching me as if they were at a charity cocktail party or entering into a highbrow business meeting, I wonder where their emotions and feelings are at. Pleasant is one thing, but over-the-top, engineered introductions (almost politician-like) become immediately interesting to me. They scream about well-defended souls; is it because of fragility or terror?

Are they self-serving or compliant? Masquerading or keeping the peace? Who is who and what is what?

My mind always goes into top gear because the first meeting gives valuable information, introducing me to initial clues about what we will be working with together; and they are usually clues to issues and traits the people cannot see for themselves. Most people presenting to me report that they have wound up in their dysfunctional and harmful position in life unknowingly, as if it crept up on them. They "had no idea" and "can't fathom it!" They "would never have guessed!"

How about when it comes to the pathological traits of NPD or codependency (CD)? No one would usually question or look behind the charming façade of an NPD-CD dance. But, there are few clues if you know what you're looking for. In fact, so well-rehearsed and fabulous is that dance that neither the perpetrator nor the victim have a clue what's going on.

But while the NPD-CD dance is the causation, the symptomatology is what really presents as painful and terrifying.

Do the following symptoms ring any bells? Loneliness in the relationship; feeling small, not respected, ridiculed, invisible, physically abused, financially extorted, emotionally abused, hooked-in and unable to move, misunderstood, unhealthy or anxious; experiencing Obsessive Compulsive Disorder (OCD); feeling deskilled, forlorn, inadequate or always wrong?

The locking in of the CD to the NPD is so complete, and has (usually) been comfortable for so long, that patients present with the symptoms above rather than bringing up a specific NPD-CD problem. In particular, for someone with NPD to see themselves as having a disorder appears to be very difficult. In fact I have never, in over 30 years of practice, had someone with NPD presenting for genuine help. However, I have had the occasional person with NPD approaching me, telling me that someone's told them that they need to get help or fix something. Really, the first thing they do is engage in a game and it's something I choose not to work with.

Codependents are usually so exhausted that they just cannot see that they are part of the dance; their most urgent need is to free themselves from all of the hooks and traps that have been set for them, but acknowledging their role as a codependent is a huge part of the healing process.

How many narcissists are out there?

According to the research I've seen from psychiatrists, 1% of people satisfy the diagnosis for NPD, with men making up three out of four cases. But the narcissist's lack of self-awareness makes it highly likely that this figure is a gross underestimate.

It is very important for me to add here that research has not sufficiently explored the same-sex and transgendered population and relies heavily on incomplete data. I have seen extreme examples of NPD in same-sex couples and in the transgendered population over the years. While I have not found the occurrence disproportionately high or low when comparing its prevalence with that in people that identify as heterosexual, the fact that there is no mention of diversity at all in the official statistics indicates that the figures may not be a complete or accurate picture.

Gatekeepers and front-line first responders, people such as myself, certainly find NPD much more prevalent than these statistics suggest and understand that it is not gender specific. In my experience, NPD respects no boundaries and can be present in any person regardless of social status, gender, age, nationality or environmental context.

Most mental health workers will tell you that narcissists are among the hardest patients to work with and are unlikely to ever seek help for themselves.

If a mental health worker being approached by a narcissist has not got the experience or understanding as to what a narcissist is, they are in for a very bumpy ride. They will be chewed up and spat out before they realise what's going on. A narcissist is an extremely intelligent, able, manipulative, cruel and grievous soul.

Opening questions

Back to our early arrivals left sitting in the waiting room. My opening expression, to bring patients into the room and encourage them to engage, is, "So what brought you to be in this room with me today?"

I leave a purposeful silence in order to allow myself time to observe and consider the body language, eye contact and other features of the dynamic.

As I am figuring out who's who in this relationship dance, I am also giving them the space to 'bring themselves.'

At the outset, I was caught from far left-field, as the man, we'll call him John, struck viciously with an outpouring of contempt for me. He didn't mess around.

He then went on, in a more pleasant manner, to explain that it was Jackie who had all the issues and that he would do anything he could to help her and her situation; a textbook example of how a narcissist will aim to sabotage therapy. He complained about how she had changed of late (they had been together for seven years) and that she no longer knew what she was doing. He explained how Jackie was getting increasingly distraught and cried "stupidly" with no reason. I asked for an example. He offered this:

It was building up to Christmas and John and Jackie had been at a supermarket.

John described Jackie's panic attack at the checkout, reporting that she had been tight-chested, unable to breathe and crying inconsolably. . . embarrassing him. At this point, Jackie moved from her hunched and frail posture and took up a forward-leaning purposeful stance. She was looking at

John from underneath a black cloud of despair—a cloud latent with irritation.

It seemed a well-practiced position. She looked as if she were exploding inside but diverting an outburst by shaking her leg violently and chewing her lips; but her eyes. . . they were fierce, at once pleading and full of rage towards John. My heart was pounding but I kept calm and remained accepting, open and inquisitive.

Throughout, John glanced at Jackie several times but seemed to not register her twisted and tormented being, as he continued to talk. As he was coming to the end of his thorough commentary of Jackie's emotional volatility, I asked him to observe Jackie and consider what was taking place with her.

Was it similar to how she was at the supermarket checkout? He affirmed that it was. He looked at me with disdain. He tried to engage with me, telling me how this was what he had to put up with.

I enquired of Jackie, "Thank you for allowing John to give me an idea of how he experiences things; now tell me what is going on for you right now?" It was as if a tap had been instantly turned on. Jackie looked to the floor, then pleadingly towards John, then I, and then back to John, and finally back to the floor.

There was a box of tissues set on the table, equidistant between John and Jackie for easy reach. Jackie did not reach for tissues and John did not offer. John looked at Jackie and then looked away, and then looked back at me and with a shrug said, "See what I mean?" Again, he was trying to convey how 'pathetic' Jackie was being.

As a practitioner, I hold back on comforting a patient in

distress, as I wish to help them engage with the discomfort and understand it as it is happening rather than extinguish the flames; this helps us to find a pathway back to the cause of distress and upset, often hidden so deeply the patient doesn't comprehend it. But how did John react? Jackie's partner of seven years seemed to show no concern or empathy, instead he ridiculed her plight.

It seemed he felt that Jackie was causing unrest and that he was the victim. Could John have an undiagnosed position? Why doesn't Jackie just leave this man?

We will return to John and Jackie later.

Narcissists are NOT in love with themselves

"Life is a stage, and when the curtain falls upon an act,
it is finished and forgotten. The emptiness of such
a life is beyond imagination."
-Alexander Lowen-

I find it is often incorrectly stated that people with NPD are in love with themselves—nothing could be further from the truth.

Looking more closely at the disorder, narcissists are out of touch with their real selves and this 'self' that they do admire—even adore—is nothing more than a fake construct, a mask behind which they can hide the terrible shame and self-loathing they feel within. Of course, hiding away behind a false mask is not peculiar to narcissists.

NPDs have found a way to use their masks to steal the energy they are unable to source for themselves from others. They are so skilled at creating this mask that they often come across as confident and charming; but this is only the handsome, well-dressed façade behind which the vampire lurks.

Far from being in love with themselves, narcissists feel chronically empty and unloved, constantly haunted by the fear of being discovered for the wretched fakes they are and the unbearable shame that would cause them.

To defend themselves, narcissists expend lots of energy controlling their appearance, behaviour and environment to extract maximum admiration by 'proving' their superiority over others.

This is what is meant by the term 'grandiosity,' one element of the antagonistic personality trait described in the DSM-5. But once the narcissist feels they are losing the floor, the mask slips and either the petulant child or the intimidating bully is likely to make an appearance. This is one of the tell-tale signs of the narcissist.

Jackie, having spent a good two minutes sobbing and taking shallow, sharp breaths, finally growled through clenched teeth at John. She explained in more detail the supermarket experience.

"We were at the checkout and John was told that one of the special offer vouchers had expired the day before. John tried to charm the checkout girl, explaining that, as a regular customer, he must have, upon this occasion, made an oversight. The checkout girl explained that the discounts were automatically deducted by the computer and there was nothing she could do.

At the same time, people in the queue behind were making comments, as our shopping was backing up. John turned from charming and smooth to rage. Red-faced and pushing me out of the way, he started to carelessly shove the shopping into bags. I reminded him that we needed to be careful as there were a few delicate gifts in one of the bags.

"John shushed me out of the way and continued to ram items in, stomping like a child—but a scary child. I felt invisible, not heard, insignificant, disrespected, not cared for—so many feelings. After years and years of this I felt I was going to explode. I just couldn't move. I pleaded with John. Once the shopping was loaded into the trolley John was polite again, thanked the check-in girl, pulled me away by my arm and told me to stop making a scene and ruining things as I always do."

Are narcissists born or made?

People often ask me what causes NPD. There is no one clear cause but there are said to be two pathways that lead there, both coming from opposite directions. One originates from the home of a child treated with cruelty. The other comes from the home of an adored child who could do no wrong.

However, there are problems with this simplistic picture. For one, sometimes this pathway instead leads to schizoid personality disorders (where the person loses their grip on reality).

Also, narcissists can exist among non-narcissistic siblings. This demonstrates that parenting alone is unlikely to be the sole cause. For the same reason, genetics cannot be the sole determinant, although various studies have provided evidence for at least an element of genetic predisposition.

For example, narcissists may be afflicted with a nervous response system that is hypersensitive to external stimuli. Combine these risk factors with a 'Western' society where individualism, competition and the creation of glamour are encouraged and you have the ideal conditions in which narcissists can flourish. In a sense, society itself has yet to develop to the stage where creating an authentic self, and learning to be comfortable with it, is the norm rather than an exception.

Looking at family history for clues
So, let's now look at John's family background and current circumstances for clues as to a possible origin.

John was brought up by parents who were quite religious. His father had worked on the railways and his mother was a stay-at-home mum with a perfectionist personality who kept everything in order. John works full-time for the local council, in a junior admin position, while Jackie is a part-time shop worker.

The couple were living together in a small, terraced house in the East End of London. Every penny they earned went towards the mortgage and general living expenses. Neither John nor Jackie had children and parenthood wasn't a priority for either of them.

The couple reported that John has a well-adjusted and successful sister who is very loving and caring. She has her own family and has been married for over a decade. John feels pressure to always be the best and is very competitive with his sister towards whom he feels great resentment. In session, John is defensive and volatile when challenged.

The problem with constructing a false ego and disowning the less palatable parts of the psyche is that people end up projecting their inner conflict onto others and creating mayhem in the world around them. In essence, this is exactly what narcissists do.

According to John, Jackie is the hysterical part of this relationship and he is the calm, collected and patient partner.

I have found that in order to keep up appearances—to themselves and others—narcissists will eventually resort to using the weapons of fear and pain, controlling those closest to them and keeping them from abandoning the relationship, because this is their worst nightmare.

Narcissists latch on to the belief that 'survival of the fittest' is the end game of existence and that any show of weakness makes them vulnerable to attack. This sets up a winner versus loser dynamic with narcissists determined to place themselves in the former category.

They, and to some extent society at large, have failed to understand that maintaining healthy boundaries while being authentic is where real strength and the desire to do good come from.

Projection

John presents Jackie as the self-obsessed 'ungrateful victim,' a clear case of a person with NPD projecting himself upon his codependent victim! Of course, if this happens daily, weekly, monthly, then the codependent's own insecurities are being deeply and dangerously affirmed.

As I mentioned before, NPD transcends gender, race, religion, sexual orientation and social status but some (inconclusive) studies have highlighted differences in how it manifests. For example, in heterosexual relationships, male narcissists tend to show the more overtly violent and controlling aspects of the disorder, perhaps helped or 'enabled' in this because women are more biologically and psychologically inclined to stay longer in an abusive relationship than is healthy.

Under this supposition, women tend to be more focused on fixing 'the one' relationship rather than looking for other opportunities, and this is intensified if she also has a passive dependent personality type, an old-fashioned psychiatric label for those who tend to become codependents.

How about NPD in same-sex couples? Although I know this exists clinically through working with same-sex couples, at the time of writing, funding has still not been applied to researching this more fully.

In my practice, I have come across no differences in the prevalence or manifestation of NPD in same-sex couples or where people with gender dysphoria (GD) are involved.

The Dark Triad

I couldn't close out this chapter without saying a few words about the so-called Dark Triad. In 2002, psychological researchers Delroy Paulhus and Kevin Williams revealed the existence of a triad of personality traits, which formed a dark core to the personality. (2)

The Dark Triad is formed from a combination of narcissism, Machiavellianism and psychopathy. These traits are on a continuum, so it is thought that everyone has them to some degree or another. The more pronounced these three traits are, the more dark and dangerous the personality becomes:

- The **narcissistic** traits give the person a sense of

entitlement and self-importance. Their needs always come first.

- The **Machiavellian** traits drive the person to plot and scheme to achieve what they want in life. They will often lie and manipulate others to do their bidding. Their first thoughts upon meeting another person entail, 'what can I get from them?

- The **psychopathic** traits remove any shreds of empathy or remorse. They also give rise to a cynicism about the motivations of other people and life in general. Psychopaths see life in evolutionary 'survival of the fittest' terms.

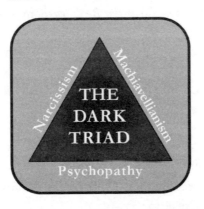

The Dark Triad theory recognises that the three traits are connected. Therefore, people with NPD are likely to also score highly on Machiavellian and psychopathic traits.

If your narcissist is particularly lacking in remorse and spends a lot of time scheming, you really need to take the message of this book seriously and plan your escape!

RECOMMENDED READING

Children of the Self-Absorbed: A Grownup's Guide to Getting Over Narcissistic Parents-Nina W. Brown

Disarming the Narcissist-Wendy Behary

Emotional Blackmail-Susan Forward

Emotional Vampires-Alan Bernstein

Malignant Self-Love: Narcissism Revisited-Sam Vaknin

The Narcissistic Family: A Guide to Diagnosis-Stephanie Pressman

Toxic Parents: Overcoming Their Hurtful Legacy and Reclaiming Your Life-Susan Forward

Trapped in the Mirror-Elan Golomb

Why Is It Always About You? The Seven Deadly Sins of Narcissism-Sandy Hotchkiss

Will I Ever Be Good Enough? Healing the Daughters of Narcissistic Mothers-Karyn McBride

"You must not hate those who do harmful things;
but with compassion, you must do what you can
to stop them—for they are harming themselves,
as well as those who suffer from their actions."
-Dalai Lama XIV-

CHAPTER 2

ENTER THE CODEPENDENT

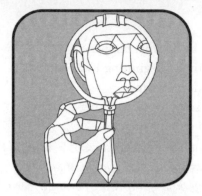

*"Look hard and deep into a mirror,
for kindness will only be reflected here."*
-Michael Padraig Acton-

These are the most common utterances I hear from patients who are victims of being in a relationship with a person with NPD.

- I feel so small.
- I am pushed down all the time.
- Self-esteem drained.
- Nothing left of me.
- Don't believe the nice things anymore.
- I'm bad.
- I'm nothing if I'm not with. . .
- Who would ever want me?
- I'm unlovable.
- Feel so much shame.

- I'm not important.
- Terrified to be alone.
- So stuck.
- Double bind: damned if I do; damned if I don't.
- People don't believe me.
- Don't know what happened.
- Well, in the beginning I was adored.
- Nobody wants me.
- Can't seem to do anything right.
- I feel I am nothing.
- I see others in love.
- So different when we are alone.
- Feel discarded.
- Others are worse off.
- Can't do anything right.
- I'm stupid and selfish.
- I feel nothing. I'm numb.

As we did at the start of the last chapter, let's look at how we can define codependency.

The term came into common usage when addiction groups such as Alcoholics Anonymous began to realise that addicts were often enabled in their harmful behaviours by their partners and other family members. Just like the addicts themselves, their partners exhibited denial and deceitful behaviour, to ensure they retained control over their own positions in the relationships; that of irreplaceable caregivers. The extent of the abusive behaviour codependents would tolerate, towards themselves and others, was observed to go far beyond what most people would agree was healthy.

But codependency is not restricted to substance addictions, and is often observed in the relationships of those with certain personality disorders, especially the Cluster B disorders such as bipolar disorder (BPD) and, of course, NPD.

In fact, codependency is *required* for narcissists to have close relationships at all and, unfortunately, they are adept at seeking out and luring codependents into their lives. They are so fearful of being alone with their despised selves that their quest for a partner becomes an obsession, which can easily masquerade as passionate love.

Although there is no specific psychiatric definition of codependency, therapists like myself are very much aware of the early life experiences that end up with people taking on that role.

For example, children who grow up in homes where addiction or abuse is ongoing—or where one or more of the caregivers are themselves narcissists—are particularly vulnerable to forming codependent relationships in the future.

In childhood, their survival and emotional wellbeing have been so wrapped up in attending to the needs of others that their own identities become dependent on them playing the martyr.

Having known only 'transactional' or conditional love, they have rarely, if ever, experienced the joy of being loved for who they are.

Codependency clues from the past
Let's now look at Jackie's background:

Jackie is a part-time shop worker and the daughter of blue-collar workers in Ireland. She has a strict Catholic background with a passive father and dominant mother. Her mother was 42 (and an immigrant) and her father was 54 when they had Jackie.

Before she dropped out, Jackie had been the first in her family to go to University; she became the 'perfect child,' angelic in every way, with polite manners and a sharp mind. Growing up, Jackie was not abused in the true sense of the word but she quickly learned that she only received approval, kindness and her mother's love when she was exceptional and faultless. So, Jackie became a pleaser to her mother and never really figured out her own needs and wants. Her mother had NPD and fed off Jackie's achievement in getting to uni, boasting about her daughter to everyone in her village.

Therefore, her mother only looked as good as Jackie did. When Jackie did not do so well or stepped off the princess perch for a moment, she was quickly punished with silence, looks of disapproval and the withdrawal of love and affection. Consequently, she developed anxiety and attachment issues and became very lonely and isolated. Jackie developed into a star codependent: 'Mother loves me when I do everything she needs. If Mother's world is OK then mine will be OK and I will be loved.'

Just like narcissists, codependents feed off the approval of others but, in their case, they define their self-worth by how well they provide for their partners. Sadly, all efforts to serve narcissists are futile as they cannot recognise nor appreciate the codependents' efforts.

Here is an example of that dynamic at play:

Jackie: "It was a Friday and we had both had busy weeks at work. I put some flowers out, baked John's favourite cake and spruced myself up. John didn't acknowledge me; he walked right past me and the flowers, and though I knew he could see the cake, he went straight into the home office. I went after him and explained what I had done. He said it was lovely but he had important things to finish and he would be with me later. I cried and he screamed at me for always making it 'about me' and said that he was tired of me ruining his evenings.

He explained the importance of this new work project, that he was tired, had just got home and that he hadn't time for any of this. I just felt that there was nothing I could do to make him feel special, that I never got it right and that I should be more understanding and not bother him. I always seem to get in the way somehow.

I'm not like this at work, only at home with John. It seems I can fool colleagues and customers at work but when people get close to me they see the real me; I just can't seem to get it right. Another ruined night and another night alone. John is busy and I must understand this."

As you can see, an NPD-codependent dynamic is a marriage made in Hell: two people locked together in a dance of mutual need, one compelled to please, the other compelled to seek admiration. Neither can exist without the other, yet true love and companionship eludes them both.

There is similarity here with domestic abuse situations because many abusers are narcissists and their victims are filling the only remaining role in a codependent relationship.

Again, it needs to be made clear that both men and women

can be diagnosed with NPD and that same-sex relationships are equally at risk of entering into this unhealthy dynamic.

Why codependents make the perfect match

Let's look deeper into the development of codependency.

Socialised to serve, the codependent's childhood need for a mother or father figure to appease is shifted onto their partner (or sibling or boss). They mistake their own desperation to please—based on a fear of rejection—for love. Just like the narcissist, the codependent has no resources for dealing with being alone.

To recover, a codependent desperately needs to work on defining what belongs to them and what belongs to others (i.e. creating boundaries). But, trapped in a relationship with a narcissist that becomes impossible because the narcissist is constantly working against that aim, eroding what few boundaries the codependent does have, so that they will tolerate a far greater level of abuse than someone with healthy boundaries. This is rarely understood by those who are outside and looking in.

From being idolised to despised

Jackie explained that she is slowly eroding away and disintegrating into the relationship, losing herself in the process.

The relationship had started with her being swept off her feet and paraded in front of John's friends, colleagues and family as smart, beautiful, amazing and special. John apparently idolised and loved Jackie and she was so happy because she had found her true love. He was such a catch too: charming, tall, handsome and well-respected by everyone.

Once they started living together, Jackie began to feel uneasy, yet at the same time comfortable, with the familiarity. It was some time before she realised the source of her discomfort: she was beginning to feel as if she had moved back in with her mother.

Because she adored and loved John, she became aware of the clues that she was trained to pick up on: that something wasn't quite right or that she needed to take care of him better (because John was 'more important than her').

Even when John's abusive and disrespectful behaviour became obvious and too much to bear, she felt she had no choice because she had nothing else. Everything was in his name, since he was the bread-winner. If she left, she would have only a suitcase and her meagre earnings from her part-time job. She was a failure as a daughter and who would want her if she failed in this relationship too?

Jackie is respected at work for her academic achievements and she has a network of close friends. But she feels worthless and 'in the way'—a waste of space—without John. You would never realise this by looking at her. She is very attractive and well-groomed. You would never, in a million years, guess what a dark sense of self she has.

John also believes Jackie has nothing without him and that he is all she needs and all she should want. He also believes Jackie is fortunate that he puts up with her at all, even though she could damage his reputation at work and with his friends if she doesn't do what's right (what he wants, in his way, when he wants it).

Jackie has been working so hard at not upsetting John—and being there to assist him—that she has neglected friends and family and isolated herself; John is really becoming all she has. Her mother taught her how to be the best people-pleaser—to her detriment.

People ask me whether the narcissist is ever moved by their codependent's efforts. Sadly, no. Any affection, attention and commitment that is showered on the narcissist never reaches past the image. No matter what their codependent does, the narcissist will eventually move the goalposts or raise the bar to ensure they fail. And as the narcissist abuses this failed self that they are projecting on to their victim, their codependent, in turn, recognises their own lack of self-love and accepts their lot.

It is a slow and gradual, but very definite, progression and a difficult phenomenon to step back from and understand. Friends and family rarely suspect a thing as all seems charming, perfect and ideal.

RECOMMENDED READING

Codependents Anonymous-CODA

Codependency for Dummies-Darlene Lancer

Codependent No More-Melody Beattie

Facing Codependence: What It Is, Where It Comes From, How It Sabotages Our Lives-Pia Mellody

Healing the Shame that Binds You-John Bradshaw

The Language of Letting Go-Melody Beattie

The New Codependent: Help and Guidance for Today's Generation-Melody Beattie

Prodependence: Moving Beyond Codependence-Robert Weiss

The Real Dope on Living With an Addict: How Addiction Saved My Life-Meredith Elliott Powell

The Road Back to Me: Healing and Recovery from Codependency, Addiction, Enabling, and Low Self Esteem-Lisa A. Romano

You're Not Crazy-You're Codependent: What Everyone Affected by Addiction, Abuse, Trauma or Toxic Shaming Must Know to Have Peace in Their Lives-Jeanette Elisabeth Menter

CHAPTER 3

EARLY SIGNS: HOW DO WE KNOW WE'VE BEEN HOOKED BY A NARCISSIST?

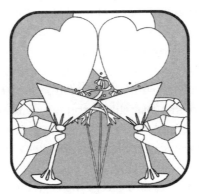

"I am living a death:
isolated and demeaned."
-Michael Padraig Acton-

Chaos and destruction

Another question I'm regularly asked is whether narcissists ever feel remorse. Narcissists are not only largely oblivious to the pain and suffering they cause to those connected with them, but they also perceive their own lack of emotional intelligence as evidence in support of their unique qualities; as a strength which lifts them above those around them.

Tragically, codependents recognise their narcissists' insecurities and put their whole beings into trying to 'fix' them. As they strive to do better and to be more worthwhile partners, parents or children, the narcissists take the opportunity to offload all of their self-hate onto their willing victims over which they begin to assert complete dominance and maintain their pathological illusion of power.

This has tragic consequences, with the tormented partners ending up more psychologically damaged the longer they stay in the situation. Their only recourse is to escape the relationship and seek therapy to help them to fully disconnect and work towards recovery.

The impact of a narcissist's abuse on those they are in a close relationship with should not be underestimated, as it affects everything that the personality is founded upon.

Very few people who have walked the corridors of my therapy rooms over the past few decades have stayed permanently with a partner who has NPD. They work hard to change themselves and accept their partner's traits but, in the end, it is usually a question of life and death—they have to get away.

The only two people I know to have continued in their relationship stepped back, recognised their situation, made a life for themselves separate from their relationship and expected very little from their partner. Both had multiple affairs but they stayed together for practical reasons, played the narcissist's required game and were fulfilled outside of the relationship. Both are in the public eye and 'for now' it serves them well to stay together. The takeaway message is: if you are in love and needing a narcissist, you are hooked. It is very hard to unhook, separate from a narcissist and live a life of convenience. The key is falling out of love, because if you fall out of love with a narcissist, you are no longer hooked!

Some of my patients have turned themselves inside out

during this work. They have examined their souls and looked deeply into the mirror—no holds barred. It really is an amazing piece of work and I have had the privilege of working at this level of intensity 50-plus times in my career.

So, how do codependents like Jackie get hooked in the first place? In the early stages of a relationship, the person with NPD is highly skilled at presenting themselves as level-headed, caring, generous and considerate. They are often so focused on obtaining the narcissistic supply only an intimate relationship can provide, that they are frighteningly skilled at quickly and powerfully sourcing a romantic partner.

The victim/codependent falls for the mask, unaware of the danger they are heading for, particularly the young and naïve who have not had the life experience or parental guidance that can save them.

The more wary person might pick up on the narcissist's Achilles' Heel, which is their insatiable need to be admired. If the attention isn't on them, the narcissist will quickly show signs of boredom, frustration and even anger.

For many others, the dream begins to unravel gradually, with the narcissist subtly increasing their power at the expense of their partner's. By the time any overt physical or psychological coercion begins, the codependent is already deeply enmeshed in the relationship: a web of destruction.

Unable to form a genuine, loving bond, the narcissist will also destroy parents, children and even work colleagues in his or her campaign for ultimate control.

Making a shift
Jackie and John approached me for couples work. John stayed

for two sessions and told me that he felt I was qualified, exceptionally experienced and really good at my job.

He told me confidently that I was the person that could help "his Jackie," because, to him, it was Jackie who desperately needed my help. It became abundantly clear that he was dumping Jackie on me 'to fix.'

After working with Jackie for a few individual sessions, we came to engaging in this dialogue, "Jackie, we have been working for a while now and I sense you are lost; it is very difficult to see *you* in the stories you are telling me. Might I pull us both back and review where we are? You have spoken about your mother, your siblings, your colleagues and John; however, through all of this I really do not know what you are here to accomplish. I feel it would be an idea to think about what Jackie needs, what Jackie wants."

There was a very long silence; Jackie looked at the floor directly in front of her feet. I kept quite still and silent and had to remind myself to breathe for I felt I had knocked the nail of the issue on the head.

Slowly, Jackie raised her head and with a soft but assertive and reflective delivery she said, "What an unusual and interesting question. What's more interesting is. . . I really don't know. My initial thought was to have John and I happy again but I realise 'want' and 'need' are very different. I need John to be happy again, but what do I want? What does Jackie want? How can I know what I want when I don't even know who I am? I DON'T KNOW WHO I AM!"

Jackie released a haunting, howling moan. Her face contorted and she visibly deflated in front of my very eyes. Jackie was making a 'shift.'

In psychological terms, she had seen her reflection and no one was there.

Jackie had been serving her mother and John her entire life; John had simply replaced her mother. She discovered that even her choice of academic degree was made to please her mother (and was perhaps the reason why she failed the course). The place where she lived with John was not her choice of home; she lived there because he liked it. She realised that there was not one picture on the wall that she had chosen or even liked; in fact, when she had expressed liking something, John had talked her out of getting it. All of this happened in the space of 10 minutes and as quickly as this outpouring had started, it stopped.

Jackie felt terrible talking about this and left the session; I didn't hear from her for a month. In fact, it wasn't Jackie I heard from next; it was John.

It starts with confusion

What are the first signs of a problem developing in a codependent relationship with a narcissist?

I find that the first symptom is often a vague feeling of confusion. The narcissist rarely unleashes his or her full pathology on their partner in one blast, revealing their flaws in small ways at first. This is a reason for one of the huge misconceptions around NPD. The fully revealed personality disorder is so monstrous, those outside the relationship fail to understand the calculated escalation that turns seemingly strong, independent individuals into helpless shells. By the time the narcissist is out of the shadows, their partner has been worn into such a state of psychological exhaustion that they are unable to form the protective boundaries that are part and parcel of a normal healthy relationship.

Following an episode of abuse, the narcissist can often disarm their victim through a twin process of carefully apportioned blame, "If you hadn't made me look so bad in front of my friends, I wouldn't have been so angry." Also, mock remorse, "I love you so much; I promise this will never happen again." The process works a treat on the codependent partner who accepts the poisoned chalice and redoubles their efforts to give the narcissist what they need.

The increased attention serves to feed the narcissist but also to repulse them, as they see their own projected neediness reflected back at them. As the unhealthy bond continues to develop and becomes embedded, verbal and physical abuse often escalates which inevitably leads to serious psychological and sometimes physical harm.

Why stay with a narcissist?

It was an extremely hot day and all of the windows were fully open. I was grateful for every breeze that came, for the room was sticky and the fan laboured to keep the air moving and the room comfortable enough for my patients and I to focus (the windows need to be closed during session because of the potential for people in the office next door to hear). I felt slightly irritable in the heat and was trying to calm myself when a call came through from John asking for my urgent help.

John reported that he and Jackie had been attending a business dinner when Jackie seemed to start suffocating, before yelling at him and leaving the restaurant. John found her outside and demanded she return and apologise. Instead, Jackie ran away, literally ran as fast as she could, and did not return home until hours later.

John emphasised how Jackie needed help and that he was counting on me to help her, as she was out of control and causing all sorts of issues for him. John also made reference to his faith in me to do a 'good job' and to get Jackie back to her 'normal' self.

He instructed me to call Jackie and arrange an appointment with her. I explained to him that it would be better if Jackie were to access me herself and acknowledge that she needs this help. He seemed irritated with this suggestion but Jackie did call.

I really wanted to ask John, if she was that much trouble, why was he still with her? Unfortunately, there was no agreement to work with John on this but it would be a very good question to ask Jackie if she were to get in touch—to turn the tables and bring in that perspective. If she is really that bad—worthless and damaging and ruining things—why was John still with her?

Recognising the warning sounds of NPD
Here follows some of the warning signs I commonly associate with narcissists:

- A lack of humility. True narcissists are 'never wrong' and never feel remorseful. Although they may apologise for a situation, this will almost always be accompanied by a thinly-disguised excuse with the victim blamed in some way.
- Since they believe they are never wrong, narcissists often react angrily when criticised.

- Narcissists are skilled at commanding the attention and admiration of others, often boasting about their achievements.
- Narcissists are so disconnected from themselves that they can't even begin to relate to others on an emotional level. Empathy and, by extension, love are alien concepts to them, although they are often able to put on an act to cover up this deficiency.
- Narcissists will often call and/or text their partners excessively. This controlling behaviour is often misconstrued as a sign of love and commitment.
- Narcissists without attention will become either sulky, depressed or angry.
- Narcissists despise normality and see themselves as above everyday concerns (which rarely provide them with the special attention they crave).
- This can mean they fail to hold down a job or handle finances responsibly, often deliberately engineering crises to direct attention onto them.

Please note here that there is a wealth of theory about, and numerous observations of, NPD behaviour. Not every box above needs to be ticked.

NPD is more about an attitude and, although there is, of course, common ground shared by narcissists, they, like all humans, are individuals. Thus, there may be exceptions to the rule and even 'typical' narcissists may show more of one trait and less of another. Regardless, everyone with NPD governs, controls and feeds on their intimate partner, child, sibling or parent to survive.

*"Believe nothing, no matter where you read it, or who said it,
no matter if I have said it, unless it agrees with your own reason
and your own common sense."*
-Buddha-

The perfect partner

Whenever I've worked with a codependent, whether they are a medical director or car salesperson, they don't want that initial six months or year, where they were swept off their feet, to have meant nothing. They felt they were really in love but they were actually prey being hooked. When it's too good to be true, it usually is. . . unfortunately. It's a difficult thing we, as therapists, have to do: recognise that people want to hold onto some beautiful memories but at the same time help them to understand how deceptive those experiences really were.

Ironically, one of the most common precursors to the narcissist-codependent relationship is the whirlwind romance that sweeps the victim off their feet. This is because the narcissist has learned to become the perfect actor. If they were to reveal their true nature at the outset of a relationship, they would quickly be tossed aside.

So they work diligently to simulate the perfect partner, keeping up this charade for many weeks or even months, before letting their real selves show through.

Too good to be true?

Although romantic gestures should be appreciated and enjoyed, people must retain some healthy scepticism, particularly if they become aware of worrying inconsistencies in behaviour. Jackie's main recurring story is about how she does not understand what went wrong—or what she did wrong—because this was her dream relationship and everyone loves and admires John.

"I just don't understand what is wrong; no matter how hard I try, I don't get it right," she told me.

One character trait that should ring alarm bells, even during the 'honeymoon period,' is a disproportionate reaction when the partner turns off the supply of attention.

Regardless of their romantic gestures and promises of love, the narcissist's real objectives are twofold: first, to feed directly off the admiration and appreciation the codependent lavishes on them. Second, to use that display of adoration, along with other aspects of their partner's appeal, to enhance their own image in the eyes of others (i.e. show off the 'trophy partner').

As long as the attention is flowing their way, they will be an absolute delight to be around and display all the charm and charisma they are capable of. But as soon as they feel they are 'losing the floor,' they are likely to rapidly change their demeanour, becoming withdrawn and sulky or irritable.

Unlike a truly self-confident person, a narcissist will become agitated and sometimes quite unpleasant if their partner provides attention to their other friends, although they will do their best to hide these feelings at first.

Those with an instinct for self-preservation will often do a bit of subtle background research on a new romantic interest before becoming too committed. By talking to a narcissist's friends and family members they are more likely to uncover inconsistencies around career, status or history. Assessing their relationship with their parents and previous romantic relationships, including how these ended, can throw up further insights, perhaps revealing a history of jealousy or violence.

While nobody's background is perfect, if the person's track record suggests a very different character to the one they are outwardly showing, it is often best to get out early.

Selfish lovemaking

Another warning sign is selfish lovemaking, especially if there is a lot of aggression and/or perversion involved. This is why it is usually best not to rush into a sexual relationship before being sure that both people are caring and considerate of each other's needs.

Jackie, "Even sex hurts; I've told John many times that we need to get warmed up and do some nice things, like we did in the beginning but now he just grabs me and it hurts. When I try to pull away he makes me pay for days with silence and by withdrawing from me. Again, I've ruined everything."

It is worth mentioning at this stage that sexual problems can be made worse by medications either partner may be taking. In particular, psychiatric drugs can mess up the hormonal balance in your brain.

It is shocking how much medication is prescribed after a consultation of between 10 minutes or an hour at most. It reinforces the message that the patient is the problem and not their relationships and environment. But that argument is best left for another day. . .

RECOMMENDED READING

Dating a Narcissist: The Brutal Truth You Don't Want to Hear-Theresa J. Covert

How to Spot a Dangerous Man Before You Get Involved-Sandra L. Brown

The Narcissist's Playbook: How to Win a Game You Never Intended to Play-Dana Morningstar

Narcissistic Lovers: How to Cope, Recover and Move On-Cynthia Zayn and Kevin Dibble

Prepare to Be Tortured: The Price You Will Pay for Dating a Narcissist-A. B. Jamieson

Red Flag: 50 Warning Signs of Narcissistic Seduction-H. G. Tudor

Sitting Target: How and Why a Narcissist Chooses You-H. G. Tudor

So You're Dating a Narcissist-Sheldon Brown

When Love is a Lie: Narcissistic Partners & the Pathological Relationship Agenda-Zari Ballard

Your Brain on Love, Sex and the Narcissist: The Biochemical Bonds that Keep Us Addicted to Our Abusers-Shahida Arabi

CHAPTER 4

THE DEVELOPMENT OF THE DYNAMIC

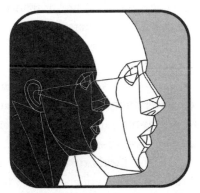

"Fake is too good to be true."
-Michael Padraig Acton-

No capacity for support
I find that one of the most shocking realisations that often confirms a narcissist's lack of empathy is their response when their partner is having a bad time and is in need of support. As the narcissist is forced to give out attention they will immediately become sulky or resentful, blaming their partner for selfishly focusing on their needs. The narcissist is actually incapable of giving out genuine warmth despite their sophisticated ability to mock concern when around other people.

For others to assert their needs is a sign of rebellion to the narcissist who may punish them for their neediness, even if they are sick. This behaviour is cruelly dehumanising and eats away at the victim's being over time.

There are no needier human beings than babies and it is interesting to note that many narcissists in a partner relationship reveal their true colours only after the birth of their first child. They simply cannot bear to lose all of that undivided attention to another person.

Chipping away over time

Seasons move so fast in the UK. I have chosen Brighton, a wonderful seaside haven in southern England, and I am sitting here listening to the far-off but loud screeches of the seagulls, as I complete the case insertions for this book.

Reflecting upon the kinds of behaviour displayed by someone with NPD towards a codependent, I find it difficult to put into words specific case examples. I've seen many codependents and helped them to unhook from their very unhealthy relationship dynamics; but there have been so many that it feels difficult to unravel them all.

However, this is probably mirroring what the codependent feels and experiences. In essence, the narcissist chips, chips, chips away at their victim over time.

The codependent knows that they have been destroyed but the main challenge is getting them to believe that the narcissist is being unreasonable and treating them unfairly.

Another challenge for the victim is to get them to give examples of the narcissist's cruelty without sounding guilty when doing so.

Jackie, for example, would often retract her complaints about John because she felt guilty or unreasonable. After all, he "gives her so much," and, "is a really nice guy, when you get to know him." Jackie oscillated between this very compassionate and loyal stance and a painful awakening about how John was and continued to be unreasonable.

Jackie's breakthrough came when she had an affair. She told me, "Michael, he is so affectionate; he touches my arm, looks at me when we are out and makes me feel really comfortable."

She once said, "He keeps telling me to stop apologising. I am realising how starved I was, all those years gobbling up any crumb of thought, kindness and affection but it felt ALL FAKE, like he was playing a role. Nothing felt like this! WHAT BROUGHT ME TO THE POINT OF FEELING I NEED TO APOLOGISE ALL THE TIME? JOHN NEVER ONCE APOLOGISED TO ME, NOT ONCE!

He's been charming and given me all the promises in the world but he was always patronising. WHY DID I NOT SEE THIS? NOTHING CHANGED! EVER!"

Jackie, by this time, was screaming and releasing pain and torment; yes, that's a good word for this: torment. Jackie was almost howling whilst engaging with all of the wrongs that had befallen her.

All of the disappointments, punishments, unfairness, loneliness, hoping, anguish and pain. It was a pain she could not put into words. It was the release of a monstrous Hell she was finally realising she needed to separate from.

This was now a case of Jackie's survival and I am not dramatising; it had got to a matter of life over death, as Jackie had planned on taking her own life if she couldn't stop the pain.

The above is what I commonly describe as a 'shift' in my therapeutic work. Jackie had worked so very hard to get to this juncture where she was finally seeing the wood for the trees.

She was realising that she had no power to change John;

she was starting to accept that the hope she had held on to for year after painful year was without grounds. The situation she was—and had always been in—was hopeless and dangerous.

The Jekyll and Hyde complex

NPD has a bipolar nature. I find that narcissists can be disarmingly pleasant and seemingly thoughtful at times, but when the weather changes, other people hardly exist to them and probably wouldn't even want to be in the same room for fear of being verbally or even physically attacked.

This can be understood when one realises that the narcissist's default state is one of emptiness. When supplied with attention from the outside world, they are satisfied, albeit temporarily, and can be good-natured to those around them. Once the supply is gone and their reserves are depleted, the negative feelings resurface, their mood crashes and the codependent finds themselves walking on eggshells again.

Behind the roar of the raging narcissist is one dominant message, "Don't damage my story and the image I have of myself and my world!"

Walking on eggshells

The conversation between myself, John and Jackie continued as follows:

John (in a suspicious tone): "Please take care of Jackie, Michael, she is not her normal self. She's becoming unbearable. I know something's up with her."

Jackie: "I cannot walk on eggshells anymore; I try to please him but what's the point? I cannot do it anymore. When he walks in front of me he gets my hand and pulls me along; I want him to hold my hand with affection, not control."

"I couldn't help it, Michael. I just broke free and ran and ran and ran. I felt that I was suffocating; I couldn't get my breath. I felt that if I didn't run. . . I don't know what."

"I ran for what seemed hours; I don't think John even ran after me, I didn't look back to check. In fact, all I remember is breaking free and running; running just to get away."

"I was gone for several hours. I sat on a park bench and just stared into space. Eventually, I got cold and had nowhere else to go, so I went home. That was the only time John ever really took notice of me and what I was doing. He demanded I sort myself out, saying that it was outrageous me leaving him in the street like that and asking if I didn't know how much he worried about me when I was gone."

Disowned feelings and projection

Do narcissists ever show a vulnerable side? Rarely, in my experience. If someone with NPD feels unfulfilled, they have no reserves on which to draw but, totally out of touch with their feelings, they will hardly ever admit that they feel 'down.'

To tarnish their fake self-image with the impurity of vulnerability is unacceptable, so they will instead start blaming those around them for making them act in certain ways. Once again, we see the hallmark of the domestic abuse perpetrator who blames the victim for 'making' them lash out due to some arbitrary departure from required behaviour. But, as there is no real match between the victim's behaviour and the perpetrator's abuse, the victim is reduced to a state of hyper-vigilance that will eventually harm both the mind and body.

Worse still, the narcissist disowns all that they despise about themselves and, through the psychological mechanism of projection, sees their inner sense of worthlessness and disgust personified in their victim. The codependent then becomes 'fair game' for any and all verbal or physical 'acting out'—an object into which the narcissist pours all of their repressed rage and hatred.

Panic attacks and safe words

I had the first couples session with John and Jackie quite far (about 14 months) into our work together. Jackie had asked to bring John in to clarify some boundary settings she felt she needed in order to continue living with him. In the session, we discussed Jackie's 'running.' Her tearing away from John and running was becoming a regular occurrence, at least twice each month.

We also looked at the situation with Jackie's panic attack at the supermarket, described in that first session. Jackie was trying to set a boundary with John whereby he hears what she says and respects her so I set the boundary that Jackie was not to interrupt John describing the events that led up to her panicking or running. In turn, I would request the same of John: that he would hear and be quiet during Jackie's recollection of events.

John: "We were at the supermarket checkout after a long day of Christmas shopping.

"There was a long queue and the weather was bad. I had bought a two-for-one offer and the receipt was wrong. The checkout girl argued with me that my voucher had expired and she couldn't do anything about it. She was disrespectful and rude.

"I told her again, in a kind way, that I was a regular customer and the voucher was only out by a day. Then people behind started to mutter and criticise because we were holding them up. It was terrible; I will never shop with them again. So, I started to pack the bags in a hurry. Next thing I know, Jackie is crying and having a panic attack."

Jackie: "Yes, the voucher had expired. I had explained this to him earlier and he had told me that since he was a regular customer it would be OK and to not be stupid. At the till, John was trying to convince the checkout girl that she could overlook just one day. He was trying to win her over by charming her. When she stuck to her guns and the people behind started to get restless, John got angry and starting packing things in bags carelessly. I explained that we would need to be careful as there were some fragile Christmas gifts I had bought earlier in some of the bags. John just gave me a warning look and continued to shove the shopping in without any consideration.

"I could see and hear that things were being smashed and broken. I—just—I—I—I felt invisible, I felt scared, I felt deflated, hopeless—I couldn't breathe!"

John, Jackie and I discussed this event at some length. John was becoming more and more agitated, as he attempted to have me side with him and see his point of view and to agree how 'silly' and unreasonable Jackie was.

I asked John if it was acceptable to seemingly ignore Jackie and break her things, to put a queue of people being frustrated before Jackie's pleading.

He eventually conceded this one point but then said to me, "So you've solved this one incident. What about the thousands of others Jackie keeps going on about? What can we do about those? How are you going to fix all of these other problems Jackie has?"

I responded that maybe we could look at how he sees things as different, to consider some boundaries, or a safe word such as 'lampshade.' Jackie could say 'lampshade' when she does not feel heard or feels threatened.

Shockingly, but expected all the same, John's guns turned on me. He exploded and accused me of being a fake, saying that he was, "tired of my advertisement to get more money from him." He added that Jackie was, "done with this stupid nonsense." And said that I was, "hurting rather than helping her." He told me that he would take me to court and sue me for every penny he had paid for Jackie plus all damages.

Soon after, Jackie came to me on her own, desperate to continue with individual therapy. I immediately drew on my funding pot to ensure she received the continuity she needed.

At our next individual session, Jackie told me how pleased she was that John had shown his 'other side.' "My friends and even family feel I'm making things up or exaggerating," she said. "John is such a charming man. No one believes me; no one gets how it is and when I try to explain it and the words come out of my mouth it sounds ridiculous, even to me. I sound like I am so ungrateful."

People ask me why narcissists like John don't simply ditch the objects of their contempt? People with NPD need attention. Although they can get a certain amount from the world at large, they still need a constant supply at home to ensure they don't have to spend time alone with themselves.

For the narcissist, the pursuit of a love partner becomes an obsession and the traits they look for are on the one hand attractiveness and status, as this enhances their own image, and, on the other hand, a poor boundary function. This will give them the purchase they need to gradually take control of the relationship–and wear down the partner's own identity.

"I just don't understand"

Jackie, we must remember, is smart and respected at work. John is very good at his admin job. Jackie's most common phrase is, "I just don't understand. When we are out, John shows me off but when we are alone it's as if I don't exist; I'm invisible. I am not like this in any other part of my world and with any other relationships, only when I'm with John. My friends and family and colleagues are great and I am liked. I just don't understand."

The child in an adult's body

The narcissist is like an angry child who has never grown up. As I explained earlier, they can emerge from families in which there was a profound lack of nurture or, conversely, those in which they were very much doted upon and 'spoilt.'

The narcissist's emotional development is arrested at around the years of five to seven and they never develop the moderating, objective part of the mind that weighs up actions and effects; this makes them exceedingly impulsive and sometimes aggressive.

Just like a child, the narcissist only really understands their own emotional pain and that becomes justification enough for any of their actions. They are intensely ego-driven and feel entitled to preferential treatment, demanding instant gratification and unable to accept being denied what they want, when they want it.

The narcissist is the archetypal con-artist and has no respect for the boundaries of others.

They are often highly intelligent and always possessed of dangerous street cunning, adept at hiding their true nature and using their acute perception and skills of analysis to select the best tactic to appeal to the emotions of their victim. In fact, the high level narcissist is supremely intuitive and manipulative, able to accurately assess weakness, rapidly move themselves into a position of trust and to begin to gather intelligence and elicit closely-guarded secrets; all used to strengthen their position.

Once accepted as a trusted partner, the narcissist lives a parasitic existence, taking what they can from their host with no consideration of the effects.

This includes money, sex and less tangible resources, such as their victim's mental focus and emotional energy. However, no matter how much is given and how often, the narcissist can never be fulfilled and will always need more.

Jackie is consistently exhausted and feels ground down, depleted, worthless and hopeless.

Some psychologists like to divide narcissists into somatic and cerebral subtypes, with the somatic narcissist requiring more of the physical and sensory supply (e.g. sex and the power that money brings) and the cerebral narcissist being more intent on lapping up attention and recognition for their intelligence and abilities.

John's most common utterance was, "I don't feel respected. I am highly regarded at work."

In a narcissist's world, all interaction is a competition where there can be only one winner; what's more, they believe other people think in the same way.

But just as in the myth of the vampire, the narcissist has to be allowed into their victim's private space before they can begin to suck them dry.

The narcissist knows that material wealth is a powerful source of attraction, and they will work diligently to create an illusion of power and self-sufficiency.

On the surface, they may display and talk about their possessions, respected role at work, nice home, car and the like.

But delve beneath the surface and all is rarely what it seems. The narcissist's sense of entitlement together with loose morals, a lack of accountability and a disdain for 'normality' will often lead them to take shortcuts and risks, and to obtain nice things by deception, the profligate use of credit and, of course, by taking advantage of the generosity of others whenever possible.

It seems that John's only value of self lies within his possessions and status at work. Has he gone into debt or borrowed from family to fund these?

It is hard to judge. While most narcissists do exaggerate and create a false image of accomplishment, their circumstances are diverse and it is important to understand that someone who has genuinely worked hard for their home and car can still be a narcissist, and they will use their possessions as a tool for self-nurturing.

The narcissist will begrudgingly do the minimum expected to fulfil their responsibilities to the 'system' while creating problems and crises around them. The true extent of the chaos in which they exist usually only becomes apparent after they have formed a powerful bond with their codependent.

In therapy, I have found that any attempt to expose the real situation is keenly felt as a wound to their self-esteem and the narcissist will react in the customary fashion of rage, denial and blame; followed by a need to boost their narcissistic supply.

Attempting to expose their hidden shame is futile; the narcissist isn't emotionally developed enough to consciously accept and process this emotion.

The green-eyed monster
The narcissist is characterised by intense jealousy, based on insecurity, and is sometimes aroused by sexual perversions. In heterosexual relationships, there is often a simultaneous obsession and hatred towards the opposite sex, which comes out verbally and physically when conflicts arise. In fact, I have found that the narcissist will often use gender-specific

slurs as they attempt to run their victim's self-esteem into the ground.

The narcissist has never learned that a relationship has to be based on trust and honesty to flourish and they will regularly lie and use dishonest tactics to gain control. Honesty is equated with vulnerability and weakness, attributes the narcissist will go to any ends to deny in themselves. The narcissist is so skilled in the art of manipulation, and so lacking in real self-awareness, that they can start to believe their own lies.

Gaslighting

Gaslighting is a psychological technique whereby an abuser, whether a narcissist or not, deliberately attempts to undermine the victim's perception of reality by doing something and then denying that 'something' has happened.

The first reference I could find for gaslighting in a psychological context was in 1978 when Martin Symonds M.D. referred to it as emotional torture and a variation of placing the victim in a double-bind.

The double-bind is that the victim has to either accept the abuser's version of events (accepting that they are mistaken) or mount a futile challenge. This may result in the abuser convincing others that the victim is mistaken. Every time the victim loses, they give up power to the abuser.

Over time, the abuser gradually becomes the arbiter of reality for as long as the relationship lasts. One of the best examples of gaslighting is from the film 'Gaslight,' from which the term derives its name.

Abusive crook Gregory embarks on a campaign to convince his wife Paula, played by Ingrid Bergman, that she is losing her mind. He takes an heirloom brooch from her bag and convinces her that she has lost it. He moves pictures and pretends she has taken them. When he goes upstairs to the attic to search for jewels, Paula hears footsteps and notices the gaslights dimming. Gregory tells her it is all in her mind. In order to accelerate his attack on Paula's sanity, he engineers an excuse to keep her away from other people.

Here is part of the script from a scene in that film:

Paula: "It began before then. The first day when I found that letter."

Gregory: "What letter?"

Paula: "From that man called Bauer, Sergis Bauer."

Gregory: "Yes, you're right. That's when it began. I can see you still. Standing there and saying, 'Look! Look at this letter!' And staring at nothing."

Paula: "What?"

Gregory: "You had nothing in your hand. . . I didn't know that about your mother."

Paula: "What about my mother?"

Gregory: "Your mother was mad. . . She died in an asylum when you were one year old."

Paula: "That's not true!"

Gregory: "Would you like to hear her symptoms? It began with her imagining things. That she heard noises, footsteps, voices. And then the voices began to speak to her. And in the end she died in an asylum with no brain at all."

Gregory's gaslighting is only exposed when Paula receives validation of her sanity from a third person; a police officer who finally helps her to bring her abuser to justice.

Codependency and hypervigilance
One of the most stressful and damaging effects of being in a relationship with a narcissist is the constant state of hyper-vigilance needed to avoid trauma. I often find that the victim is constantly in a heightened state of threat-detection, always ready to react to the next outburst or attack.

The problem is that the narcissist's mood is unpredictable and connected with their own warped inner reality rather than external circumstances. This leaves the victim perpetually in a state of uncertainty, never able to fully relax.

In the field of behavioural psychology, hypervigilance has been observed in rats.

When rewards are consistently accompanied by a green light, rats will display relaxed behaviour, but when these two events are disconnected (i.e. the rewards are given at random), the rats display repetitive, compulsive behaviour.

Fight or flight
Running, running, running. Jackie's 'running' is a behaviour

related to high anxiety in a stressed environment. When we experience extreme levels of anxiety, our bodies revert back to what was needed to survive prior to our 21st century civilisation. Before our modern world, we largely became stressed because there was a physical threat to us from competitive villagers or animals. When faced with such imminent threat we either 'fight' our way out of it or we choose 'flight' and run for the hills. This is commonly known as the fight or flight mechanism.

Jackie's running is her way of managing the threat and escaping from it, thereby reducing her anxiety to a more manageable level.

Interestingly, because we run and fight better with an empty stomach and bladder, under extreme stress it's usual for us to vomit and/or experience diarrhoea. Jackie has been suffering with symptoms that are now known as Irritable Bowel Syndrome (IBS) which is often associated with stress.

The toxic effects of hypervigilance on the body and brain should not be underestimated, as large amounts of stress chemicals, for example cortisone, have been shown to damage brain tissue. The codependent in a relationship with a narcissist may become steadily more confused and their thinking increasingly deranged until total breakdown occurs.

The effects can be magnified by gaslighting, of course. For example, the narcissist might move their victim's car keys to convince them they have mislaid them or pretend a conversation progressed differently to the way the victim remembered it, even enlisting the help of allies to back up their version of events. The more 'unsure' of their own mind the codependent becomes, the more control the narcissist can take.

Other tricks favoured by the narcissist include constantly switching their preferences so that the codependent can never make the right choice and steadfastly refusing to carry out the most basic of their expected duties giving the codependent an uneven share of domestic work, grinding them down further.

Jackie carries out all duties in the home, even when she has worked at the shop all day and John has been off work! John never even clears the table after dinner or helps to load the dishwasher. When Jackie complains about this John would often see her as needy.

Eventually, the codependent, broken of all means of rebellion, may start to display symptoms of a phenomenon known as Stockholm Complex or 'capture-bonding.' They become sympathetic with their abuser, taking on their opinions and blaming themselves for their situation.

In essence, they become the perfect projection of what the narcissist hates about him or herself. This can lead to an intensification of the abuse. This is probably the main reason why victims find it difficult to leave or unhook from their NPD partner. They become so lost and out of the loop of their own reality.

The narcissistic parent

Suffice to say, healthy parenting does not come naturally to a narcissist and I find it heart-breaking to see the effect that NPD has on children.

Whereas the majority of loving parents shower attention and

affection on their children just for being alive, the narcissist sees their offspring as either a source of competition or an extension of themselves. To the narcissistic parent, their child is only of value when they bring positive attention to the narcissist themselves.

This naturally leads to the formation of a narcissistic-codependent relationship, as the child puts all of their life energy into pleasing that parent. It is a futile bid to earn the love and affection they deserve as a birth right.

One of the saddest examples I've read about in the media is that of the actress Natalie Wood and her mother Maria Zakharenko.

Russian exile Zakharenko often demonstrated the grandiosity associated with narcissists. Despite being the daughter of a business owner, she claimed she was royalty and always thought she was destined to become an actress and ballet dancer.

Her dreams never came to fruition but when a psychic predicted that her second daughter would become famous, she started to pursue her thwarted ambitions through Natalie instead.

While the level of control and micromanagement Maria exercised over her daughter would not be unique to mothers with NPD, there are numerous examples of how she used brutal, heartless tactics to embed Natalie into the Hollywood culture. She was clearly determined to bring her own dreams to life regardless of the nightmare her daughter would be forced to experience.

Here are some examples of the lack of empathy Maria showed as she groomed her daughter for stardom according to publicly available media articles:

- Natalie was trained by her mother to please the powerful men in her life from day one. At the age of five, she was placed on the lap of film director Irving Pichel and told to "make him love you."
- When Natalie was unable to summon tears for an emotional scene, Maria captured a butterfly and tore it apart in front of her daughter's eyes.
- As a 15-year-old, Maria dressed her daughter in sexy clothes in order to appeal to the 38-year-old Frank Sinatra.
- A year later, Natalie was brutally raped by a producer-actor after being invited for an audition. Her mother allegedly ordered her not to report the assault as she was not to cross powerful movie stars.

In an interesting postscript, Zakharenko had also been told by the psychic that she would die "in dark water." Zakharenko passed that fear on to her daughter who clearly suffered from aquaphobia throughout her career.

While her mother actually died from pneumonia, Wood herself drowned in 1981 while on a boating trip with her husband Robert Wagner. Had her mother's parasitic, vampiric activity been so successful that Natalie had become a codependent shell for her mother's ego? Was the chilling prediction right after all?

Co-parenting with a narcissist: a case study

Whether you're living with a narcissistic co-parent or you are divorced and rearing a child with them, the experience is lonely; it rips you apart.

From my case files, I recall the story of a woman who was

in a co-parenting arrangement with a narcissistic husband from whom she was estranged.

I was delighted when she agreed to be interviewed for a case study for this book. Here's her story:

I remember driving 240 miles to my daughter's father's house to collect her for a month.

We had decided to have my daughter live with her father because I was the only breadwinner and had needed to relocate to keep my job. Since there was a support system where my daughter and her father were living, we agreed it would be best all round; not that we had a real choice.

He never worked and always blamed everyone else for his failings. He never finished college and blamed everyone else for that too. It took his parents 19 years to conceive him and they could only have one so they idealised him.

They never saw any bad in him. Now I have learned about NPD, I can see how a horrific childhood, or an over-indulged one, can create a narcissist.

His parents even blamed our daughter as the reason he struggled so much. To them, she was the root of all his issues!

On this occasion, I had organised holiday time and family to help babysit, I had taken leave off work, I had done everything. Halfway there I called—and this was a time when there were no cellphones—and said, "I'm on schedule" and he replied, "Well, you can't have her."

This wasn't the first time, this wasn't the fifth time, this wasn't the tenth time. Ordinarily, I would have to beg and ask, "What can I do?" He would invariably ask me for more money or it could be that I needed to have her longer or I needed to pay for a holiday.

This time I just said, "I am coming and I am going to have her." So I continued driving and I was crying at the wheel, feeling very lonely.

The situation was embarrassing so I didn't tell anybody except a close friend at uni and even then I didn't reveal the extent of it.

I was so scared of what I might do to rightfully get my daughter that I called the police and asked them to accompany me to collect her. They said they couldn't attend but they took note of the address and told me that I could remove the child because we had joint custody.

But if I were hit, punched, thrown around, pushed up against the car or anything else, I was not to retaliate. I was to call the police at the safest time.

I got to the house. I knocked and he asked me in. He wanted me to stay and said I could take my daughter the next day. I was tired, having worked all day and then driven down, so I agreed. It then got into a situation where we had sex because I knew if I kept on his good side, I could probably leave with no issues.

But the next day, while I was leaving, there was drama. Everything had been fine. It was, "You're going to go off and have a nice day with mummy," and "See you soon." But just as we were driving away, he ran up to the car, shouting. I couldn't work out what he was ranting about so I just put my foot down on that accelerator pedal and got away.

There was no follow up, nothing. He didn't even enquire after her.

We had a really good time and it got to the point of bringing her back but he didn't want her.

So, I then had to reshuffle work and friends, while all the time thinking I was the bad one. He always treated me in such a manipulative way. I always felt that I was to blame for being inconvenient, not giving enough money or not doing enough caregiving.

It got worse. My new partner and I were going to America, to Disney World, and to see our family. We had the tickets, everything was booked but, a few days beforehand, we were told that my daughter could only go if we brought her father along too.

I said, "Are you crazy, that's not going to work, what do you mean?" For the first time, he couldn't manipulate the situation so he just said, "She's not going!" Because I couldn't take my daughter out of the country without express permission (otherwise it could be viewed as kidnapping) we went without her. Can you imagine how a child looking forward to a Disney trip would feel?

And it gets even worse. My daughter had been living with me on and off for a couple of years because her dad's behaviour had descended into more drinking and debt. I tried to help by lending him half of my university fees I had saved by working overseas. He promised to pay them back over six monthly instalments and thanked me. He was very good with my daughter being with me and everything seemed to be OK.

I had given him six paying-in slips (at the time there was no such thing as a bank transfer) and about a month afterwards I told him that it seemed nothing had gone in. A couple of weeks later, I said, "It's getting awkward because my fees are due in a couple of months' time."

This was received with a laugh, a real haunting laugh, and he mocked me, saying, "You didn't think you were really going to get the money back, did you?"

After that, I was having my daughter more and more and then the most shocking thing of all happened, when I found out about his court appearance!

He had been arrested because not only had his dad and I been supporting him with money but he had been working as a teacher in a school and claiming full Social Security and housing benefit at the same time. It finally caught up with him to the tune of £27,000. He has a middle-class standing and is from a good family so when I caught wind of this, I grabbed my daughter immediately and we left because I didn't want her exposed to any of it.

I was doing my doctorate when I heard the news, from his partner, that he had been taken to prison immediately and had to serve the full time in prison. This meant I automatically got full custody.

Not only did he blame me but when my daughter and I went to his home town, outside every newsagents and on the front of every local newspaper were stories about how I, the wife, had caused him to go to prison.

I tried to protect my daughter from it all but she just couldn't be shielded and had to go through a Social Services discussion about her welfare and wellbeing. It took place without me but she told them, "My mum's always been there. She's always looked after my dad and I, financially and every other way."

At the co-parent's mother's funeral, I also got another kick in the teeth. I found out that when I had struggled to buy him a car so that he could take my daughter to a school in a good area (that I was also paying for), he had actually got his father to buy the car and spent my money on ludicrous things.

So, they were very interesting times and it took me 34 years and a therapist to bring some reality and reveal to me that I had been overcompensating for my own childhood. It took that long to unhook, feeling that I was the terrible one, even though people were saying, "Oh, you're great, how terrible that this is happening to you!" It was my inner world that had created the horrific belief that I was causing all the bad things. That's what narcissists do! They trick us.

My saving grace is that whatever happened, I never allowed it to have any impact from me on my daughter. However, her father had trained her well to perform in two worlds: one, in which you're nice to somebody to get what you need and another in which you berate them or deceive them. He would even tell her what things to steal from me (DVDs, money, ornaments, etc.)

I was standing in a school playground when I finally said goodbye to this co-parent and I never intend on seeing him or talking to him ever again. The whole thing seems a blur now but some things do stay and haunt me. I wish I knew then what I know now. I would have chanced it and run away with my daughter to save us both from it all.

Narcissists look for soft touches. They look for codependents and they look for kind, concerned and reasonable people. Although this woman was doing well career-wise and every other aspect of her life was great, that one relationship almost killed her!

The death of the narcissist

I find that people often pity the lot of the narcissist and I can see why: the life of a narcissist is indeed tragic. But the way in which they can and will drag anyone they bond with into their nightmare means that sympathy is a very risky attitude to take. To the narcissist, sympathy is just another form of attention, and they will gladly lap it up until their victims have no more to give.

Underneath the mask lives a frightened and angry child, afraid of being abandoned and ignored and desperate to replace those feelings with the drugs of physical pleasure, admiration and attention. Other people exist solely to gratify these needs and are, in their eyes, little more than objects with no right to their own feelings or motivations.

Sadly, as the narcissist begins to age, they lose some of their physical appeal while, at the same time, their history of cruelty and dishonesty usually begins to catch up with them.

They may end up profoundly alone and destroyed by debt, with nowhere left to go to escape from the inner darkness they have been running from for so long.

Perhaps they will, at last, face a final reconciliation with their shadow but that is unlikely to occur in a therapist's rooms.

In all my years of practice, I have never seen a recovered narcissist.

RECOMMENDED READING

30 Covert Emotional Manipulation Tactics: How Manipulators Take Control in Personal Relationships-Adelyn Birch

The Covert Passive-Aggressive Narcissist-Debbie Mirza

From Charm to Harm: And Everything Else in Between With a Narcissist-Gregory Zaffuto

Gaslighting, Love Bombing and Flying Monkeys-Angela Atkinson

In Sheep's Clothing: Understanding and Dealing with Manipulative People-George Simon Jr.

Magic Words: How to Get What You Want from a Narcissist-Lindsey Ellison

Object of My Affection is in My Reflection: Coping with Narcissists-Rokelle Lerner

You Might Be a Narcissist If. . .: How to Identify Narcissism in Ourselves and Others and What We Can Do About It-Cynthia Munz, Lisa Charlebois and Paul Meier

The Wizard of Oz and Other Narcissists-Eleanor Payson

Web of Lies-My Life with a Narcissist-Sarah Tate

CHAPTER 5

NARCISSISM AND CODEPENDENCY IN POPULAR CULTURE

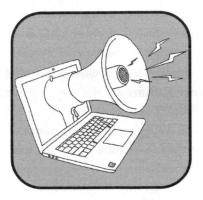

"Narcissism is not our modern day voice feeling entitled."
-Michael Padraig Acton-

There has been an explosion of interest in narcissism and codependency over the last few years. Since I published my first book, Narcissism and Codependency, new ways of talking about both conditions have entered the common language and some older terms have been revived. Everyone and their dog now has an opinion on narcissism and codependency. Some people are diagnosing fellow humans with serious psychiatric disorders because of a comment they once made on Twitter!

What is the reason for this? As I mentioned in the introduction, the drugs companies are looking for ways to manage as many people as possible through medication; the more people that are sick, the better!

The media outlets stand to profit from anything that turns ordinary lives into dramas.

There are also plenty of experts who like to add personal kudos and boost their YouTube viewing figures or search engine rankings. They do this by adding terms like 'sociopath' and 'malignant' to their diagnoses or blending disorders as if there were a psychiatric pick 'n' mix.

Whatever the reasons, the result has been a muddying of the waters with the terms narcissism, codependency and their variants bandied around whenever we want to disparage a person (Donald Trump?) or create a drama.

What about those unhappy, confused souls desperate for help?

Perhaps they gain some control over their personal pain by trying to give it a name—even if the slipper doesn't really fit.

This is why it is important that individuals, couples and families source help from the therapists with personal experience. Those who live and breathe relationship problems personally—on a daily basis—not the non-therapeutic models used by the drugs companies and psychiatrists; nor the exotic definitions given by YouTube gurus and sensation-seeking media companies.

Having said all that, to navigate this complex and shifting world, it does help to try and pin down some of those psych buzzwords and see how they fit with the reality of what therapists, such as myself, deal with in our rooms.

With that in mind, I will summarise some of the commonly-used terms and follow this with a closer look at some of the trending topics around narcissism and codependency.

Top 10 narcissism buzzwords

1. Malignant narcissism

This is a revival of a term created in the 1960s and made popular in the 1980s and 1990s by the psychoanalyst Otto Kernberg. It was originally based on the theory of a spectrum of unhealthy narcissism leading from the patient with NPD at the mild end to the psychopath at the severe end. The malignant narcissist sits between the two. The term is applied more broadly today.

2. Narcissistic sociopath

We know from the movies that sociopaths are remorseless killers so combining narcissism with sociopathy (whether as a narcissistic sociopath or sociopathic narcissist) adds an element of 'wickedness' to the definition. In truth, all sociopaths are narcissistic so why the extra ingredient? It's like talking about jam pectin or egg protein.

3. Narcissistic Borderline Personality Disorder (BPD)

Narcissistic BPD doesn't officially exist because both disorders are diagnosed separately in the DSM-5. However, there can be an overlap in traits (e.g. both can feel entitled, display rage when rejected and engage in seductive behaviours). At the end of the day, if the person you are concerned about displays the narcissistic traits detailed in this book, does it matter whether they are a pure narcissist?

4. Grandiose Personality Disorder (GPD)

The unofficial term GPD is sometimes used to separate out 'true' narcissists from those who are less obviously egotistical.

It might also be used as a colourful description by the media (e.g. the term was applied by a New York magazine writer when 'diagnosing' photographer Annie Leibovitz). Either way, it is of no use to a suffering codependent. Someone with GPD is a narcissist—pure and simple!

5.   Group/collective narcissism
Imagine a narcissist becomes the CEO of a company. They bring in people they know will do what is asked of them. The wider team, anxious to please the boss, won't allow any negative feedback to make its way to the top. Beneath the healthy façade, the company rots away until one day it sinks without trace.

6.   Narcissistic Personality Syndrome
Narcissistic Personality Syndrome is just another name for Narcissistic Personality Disorder (a syndrome is a disorder characterised by a group of symptoms which occur together).

7.   Classic/grandiose narcissist
Researchers may refer to a classic or grandiose narcissist when looking to separate out other types of narcissist. Refining diagnoses means more customised meds can be created. This distinction shouldn't concern suffering codependents. Do you see a pattern here?

The next three buzzwords are also not fully recognised by the field but have more kudos due to the work of American psychologist Theodore Millon. In 1969, Millon proposed four subtypes of narcissism (there was also a fifth 'normal' subtype). The unprincipled narcissist is similar to the malignant narcissist, so we don't need to dwell on this subtype. However, the other three are worth touching on.

8. Compensatory/covert narcissist

Millon's compensatory narcissist (sometimes called a covert narcissist) has some of the traits associated with Avoidant Personality Disorder (AvPD) namely the tendency to run away from those who threaten their identity. They therefore play out their narcissistic tendencies in fantasies and may use passive-aggressive tactics to punish others rather than confronting them directly.

9. Amorous narcissist

As the name suggests, the amorous narcissist plays out their need for attention in the romantic arena. They use their charm and seductive skills to beguile others before moving on to their next target once the flame fades.

10. Elitist narcissist

The elitist narcissist self identifies as part of an exclusive club despite having done nothing to qualify. They often form relationships with genuine high-fliers to feed off their achievements.

Malignant narcissism: the quintessence of evil?

Malignant narcissism was first defined by social psychologist Erich Fromm in 1964. He defined it as the 'quintessence of evil.'

Professor Otto Kernberg, a psychoanalyst widely known for his theories on narcissism, claimed in 1989 that there was a spectrum of unhealthy narcissism that stretched from NPD on the low end to psychopathy at the other.

According to him, the inner voice most of us have is totally lacking in the psychopath, so they don't even realise they are doing wrong when they hurt someone.

At the other end of the scale, the person with NPD has developed a very critical inner self—one that nobody, the codependent included—will ever satisfy.

Between the two—and containing the worst elements of both—is the malignant narcissist who uses cruelty as a way to achieve power over others. This sadism worsens as their inner voice becomes more warped over time. Eventually, they become closer in nature to the true psychopath.

The term malignant narcissist is used more liberally today.

Kernberg's malignant narcissist was a hopeless case, leading to progressively cruel and sadistic acts. Today, the term is used to apply to narcissists further down his spectrum—those who might lie, cheat and even kill, yet still retain a shred of remorse.

The narcissistic sociopath

What is a sociopath? It depends on what you read or who you listen to. Some treat sociopaths and psychopaths as different in name only (with those favouring social causes using the term sociopath and those favouring individual causes using the term psychopath). Others assert that the disorders follow different pathways (psychopaths are born and sociopaths made).

Yet others draw a clear distinction saying that psychopaths are sick while sociopaths are relatively normal but follow a different moral code to the rest of us.

Given that fuzzy starting point, it is hardly surprising that the term 'narcissistic sociopath' is of little use to people suffering at the hands of a narcissist.

Narcissists lack empathy, blame others for their unhappiness and have the capacity to hurt without feeling bad about it.

That's damaging enough!

Spending your time trying to decide whether you are being hurt by a narcissistic sociopath or just a 'garden variety' narcissist is like worrying about whether your head is in the jaws of a lion or a tiger!

NPD, BPD or both? Untying the knot

The fact that so many people are talking about borderline narcissists and narcissistic borderline personality disorder (BPD) sufferers serves to highlight the difficulty in teasing apart the symptoms of these disorders to get to the person beneath them.

Let's simplify this.

Borderline patients tend to present as emotionally unstable. One day they can walk into the room and be light and carefree. The next they can be ravaged by insecurity. On session three they might walk into the room with as dismissive an air as the most grandiose narcissist. Their identity is constantly in flux. They don't know who they are.

Narcissists know exactly who they are (at least, they think they do). They are tricky characters and rarely present as stereotypical narcissists—at first. In fact, they can be quite charming and the inexperienced therapist can find themselves dangerously falling for their wiles.

However, they will turn like the wind once their self-image

is challenged. Is this a mood swing? Absolutely! But it comes from a different place than BPD.

Can you see now why I argue that doctors shouldn't be diagnosing people after 10-minute consults?

If you ignore the labels and focus on the narcissistic behaviours you will find it easier to relate to the advice in this book—and take the firm and decisive action required to save yourself.

Let's take a breath. . .
If you are finding yourself scrabbling around between definitions, I recommend taking a pressing pause and going back to basics.

Narcissism has been with us since Ancient Greek times and NPD is well understood and recognised by experienced and qualified therapists.

The narcissist's false image is bolstered by the attention received from others.

Without the burden of empathy, the narcissists have learnt how to become whippet-smart, master manipulators to hook those who will give them the attention they need.

To a codependent, a narcissist becomes a parasite, relying on their host to 'feed' their illusions of grandeur. Yet, they never become satiated. Worse, they cope with their inner self-hatred by turning it outwards onto those they are feeding on.

Whether they are hurting you, seducing you, dismissing you or ignoring you, the narcissist's behaviour springs from the same root cause: a damaged sense of self. And it's a self that the codependent can only prop up—never repair.

Top 10 codependency buzzwords

1. Enabler

An enabler, in a psychological context, is someone who helps another to continue their destructive behaviour. Narcissistic control and the enabling of that behaviour by the codependent are at the core of the destructive relationship.

2. Dependent personality

There is an important distinction between codependent and dependent behaviour, which alters the whole dynamic when it comes to a relationship with a narcissist.

The dependent person primarily wants to be cared for, while the codependent wants to be the source of care. Since the narcissist and dependent are both takers they are like similar poles of a magnet. They repel. The relationship never lasts.

3. Codependent personality disorder

Codependent personality disorder doesn't exist as a psychiatric condition. . . yet!

Mental health experts have battled for decades over whether codependency needs its own 'box' in the DSM. You can be sure that those who think it should will finally get their wish once the drug companies develop a 'codependency pill.'

4. Toxic codependency

Popular sources of psychological information may try to draw a distinction between 'healthy' codependence, where the codependent's behaviours do not cause dysfunction, and toxic codependency, where they do. When a codependent is in a relationship with a narcissist, the result is ALWAYS toxic!

5. Co-addict

A co-addict is someone who enables an addict's destructive behaviour by covering up for them, making excuses for them and placing themselves as the only person who understands and can help the addict.

This term is normally reserved for the friends, partners and family members of alcoholics and drug addicts but fits equally well into the narcissist-codependent dynamic. The codependent mistakenly thinks that they can change the narcissist through their hard work and care. They are as addicted to the dysfunctional relationship as the narcissist themselves.

6. Codependency anxiety

Codependency anxiety is that sweat-drenching fear that the codependent feels at the mere thought of being abandoned by the narcissist. It is part of the engine that keeps the cycle going.

7. Codependency depression

While codependency depression is rarely discussed, many people are concerned about the effects of codependency on mental health. As the codependent begins to realise that their efforts will never bring back the perfect relationship they thought they once had, they become stuck—unfulfilled but too afraid to leave.

8. Active codependent

Therapist and author Ross Rosenborg has sought to divide codependents into two subtypes: active and passive.

The active codependent is not afraid to stand up to the narcissist and to lie and cheat to meet their own needs. They are often mistaken for narcissists but the hard work they put into changing the narcissist belies their true nature.

9. Passive codependent

In Rosenborg's theory, the passive codependent more closely fits the stereotype of the meek, subservient enabler.

10. Codependent anger

Even the codependent can only take so much before the resentment they feel within boils over. This can erupt into a violent outburst or may be directed into malicious acts of revenge. Sadly, the anger is no release. Instead, it fuels an agonising guilt at letting the narcissist down. The pattern continues with the codependent promising to 'do better' next time.

10 common enabling behaviours

Are you enabling a narcissist? It can be difficult to separate out genuine love and care for our partners, families and friends from an unhealthy pattern of self-abusive enabling.

Here are 10 behaviours often associated with enabling:

1. Coming to the rescue

Do you find yourself taking steps to save the narcissist from the consequences of their actions? For example, do you call work for the narcissist and pretend they are ill when they decide not to go in?

2. Over-functioning
Do you take on more than half of the household chores? Do you take up the slack left by the narcissist?

3. Forming a buffer
Do you control access to the narcissist (e.g. always answering the door or telephone) so you can manage their exposure to other people?

4. Endurance
Do you drive yourself forward regardless of how hard your life is? Do you believe you need to work harder at your relationship to make the narcissist happy?

5. Denial
Do you dismiss people's concerns about your relationship? Do you go out of your way to prove you are not codependent and that the person mistreating you is not a narcissist?

6. Infantilise
Do you treat the narcissist as someone who needs looking after and protecting from the reality of life?

7. Bottled emotions
Do you rarely feel able to vent your emotions? Does anger and resentment bubble below the surface? When you do emote, do the feelings erupt violently?

8.   Controlling behaviour
Are you obsessed with maintaining control of the narcissist in your life? Do you feel anxious when they ignore your requests or demands?

9.   Leniency
Are you always ready to forgive the narcissist's behaviour no matter how out of order? Do you tell yourself that their actions are down to stress or your failings and that they are nice people underneath?

10. Avoidance
Do you back down from discussing delicate topics with the narcissist? Do you feel you are walking on eggshells and it is better to keep the peace?

A people-pleaser. . . or a pleasant person?
The results of peoples' kindness in the world are often seen as problematic. When living in a society that poorly rewards the good in people, genuinely kind people are often forced to adopt coping mechanisms, such as people-pleasing, to cope with their toxic environment.

Oftentimes, people see these frustrated people-pleasers as being a 'problem' rather than the underlying 'pleasant people' they are.

So, here's to all of us 'problems'. May this book help others to understand our souls and see reason.

As one of my patients, Nicky, eloquently puts it, *"The result of my kindness not being recognised or appreciated has made me out to be 'the quiet one', 'the moody one', the one that gets walked over.*

"Me being kind in the strict overpowering environment I was bought up in has led me to adopt many coping mechanisms.

"All you see is me as a child that is out of control and not the kind, loving person I want to be.

"May you now see me as an adult, free to make my own choices, which would include, by my choice, being kind to you."

Am I dependent or codependent?

The difference between being dependent and being codependent often causes confusion. This section aims to clear the fog once and for all.

Dependency (which becomes Dependent Personality Disorder when it starts affecting the ability to function in life) affects relationships with other people in general.

Codependency (which, as yet, doesn't have an academically accepted disorder—despite therapists like me experiencing it day in, day out) affects a specific relationship.

That is the most striking difference between the conditions.

In our case study, Jackie says, "I am not like this in any other part of my world. . . only when I'm with John."

Another key difference between the two conditions is that the dependent person will make others responsible for their happiness. If they don't receive the care and attention they want, it's the other who is generally blamed.

If a codependent person doesn't receive care and attention from the person they are fixated on, they will blame themselves. As time goes on, their perception of themselves will become more warped and their self-esteem trashed.

Worse still, the codependent will become gradually more ensnared over time—it's like they're trying to wriggle out of quicksand. The dependent person, full of blame, will be quickly dumped by the narcissist—and they will be all the better off for it!

Codependent Personality Disorder: the invisible diagnosis

Patient: "Doctor, Doctor, I feel like I'm invisible."
Doctor: "Next please."

This common 'Doctor, Doctor' joke could easily have been written with the codependent in mind. Since the 1980s, those who recognise codependency as a unique disorder have argued for its inclusion in the psychiatrists' bible—the DSM.

Others argue there is too much overlap between codependency and Dependent Personality Disorder, Borderline Personality Disorder, Histrionic Personality Disorder and even Post-Traumatic Stress Disorder. They say there is simply no justification to create a separate category.

However, research since the publication of the DSM-5 has revealed cases of codependency where there has been no other diagnosable disorder. Maybe a future edition of the DSM will finally give codependents the recognition they deserve. Until then, Codependency Personality Disorder will remain an invisible illness.

In some ways, the fact that Codependency Personality Disorder isn't in the DSM-5 may be a blessing in disguise. The worst thing that could happen to a struggling codependent is for them to be prescribed 'codependency pills' and sent on their way after a 10-minute consult. What better evidence for the narcissist to say, 'there you go, it is all in your mind,' and the codependent to respond, 'I guess you're right, I'll take the pills and see if that makes me a better lover/son/daughter/mum/employee'.

Dangerous narcissists of the last century

If anyone ever doubted the seriousness of NPD in our world, my hope is that the following section challenges this! We hope this book puts NPD on the map of crimes and criminals. From cold-hearted killers and predatory paedophiles to audacious Wall Street fraudsters, here are a few of the most dangerous narcissistic criminals in history, many of whom were clinically-diagnosed NPDs:

1. Bernie Madoff
So great was his need to be admired that stock broker and investment manager Bernie Madoff systematically defrauded wealthy friends and charities through the largest pyramid scheme in world history. He has shown no real remorse for his actions.

2. Jimmy Savile
For many, the outlandish DJ and television presenter was a symbol of English eccentricity. But beneath the surface was a self-centred, manipulative, remorseless abuser and paedophile who preyed on children both inside and outside of hospitals he patroned.

3. Brian Blackwell
What turns a high-performing young man from a well-to-do

family into a brutal killer without remorse? In extreme cases, a narcissist will do anything to defend their fantasy world from being destroyed.

4. Anders Breivik

Norwegian mass murderer Anders Breivik may be portrayed as a right-wing extremist but did narcissism play a big role in fuelling his rage against the world and his lack of remorse for his actions?

5. Ted Bundy

Serial killer Ted Bundy displayed all the elements of the deadly dark triad, enabling him to charm, trap and then mercilessly destroy his female victims without a shred of remorse.

6. Diane Downs

We may never know exactly why Downs staged a car-jacking and shot her three children, killing one of them. In true NPD fashion, she has never shown remorse and created elaborate fantasies of one day escaping prison.

7. Antoinette Frank

Despite failing a psychiatric evaluation, the 'shallow and superficial' Antoinette Frank was recruited by the New Orleans police force. She went on to murder three people in a chilling armed robbery at a restaurant. The remorseless killer was rewarded with a spot on Death Row!

8. Josef Mengele

What happens when a narcissistic psychopath with a fanatical ideology and dedication to duty is given power in a murderous regime? The answer is Josef Mengele, Auschwitz's 'Angel of Death.' Mengele was capable of the most hideous of crimes and never expressed any remorse.

9. Barry Minkow

Minkow's 'ZZZZ Best' insurance restoration scam sucked in investors and funded his lavish lifestyle of sports cars and luxury mansions. He then became a pastor and defrauded his own church. Again, he showed no remorse for his crimes.

10. O.J. Simpson

The O.J. Simpson murder trial was one of the highest-profile criminal cases of the 20th century. Simpson displayed many of the traits of a narcissist including a love of the spotlight, sense of entitlement, tendency to blame others and lack of remorse.

Plus one: RR, The Black Widow

Of course, only a minority of narcissists become convicted killers or billion-dollar con artists. However, that should not take away from the heartbreak and chaos that a committed NPD can unleash once they are latched on to their victims.

You will soon read, in Chapter 6, about a case of NPD I have been heavily involved with. I truly believe that, given the opportunity, RR, the Black Widow, is capable of some of the heartless acts mentioned above. She would certainly strip the wealth from millionaires and billionaires without blinking an eye or feeling any shred of remorse. Could she kill to keep her fantasies alive? I hope that I never find out!

Bernie Madoff: the wizard of lies

The scale of Bernie Madoff's US$64 billion fraud was so stunning that his story made its way on to the silver screen as *The Wizard of Lies,* with Robert De Niro playing the part of Bernie and Michelle Pfeiffer starring as his long-suffering wife, Ruth.

Is Madoff a narcissist? He certainly ticks most of the boxes. High-performing narcissists always aim for the top, a position they feel is their natural destiny. As chairman of his own company, Bernie L. Madoff Investment Securities LLC, Madoff sat literally at the summit of the world's biggest-ever pyramid scheme. After his company helped to develop its foundational technology, Madoff also became non-executive chairman of the NASDAQ stock exchange.

But it is what he did to get there that truly marks him out as a narcissist. Not only do narcissists lack empathy, they also often act with disregard for the consequences of their actions.

Madoff didn't just rip off faceless investors. He deliberately and systematically reeled in wealthy friends and associates and, over decades, defrauded them of billions of dollars.

Worst of all, Madoff heartlessly stripped many charitable foundations and hospitals of their assets, causing some to shut down. Shamelessly, he even exploited his own flesh and blood, only admitting to his sons (whom he employed) that the whole Ponzi scheme was a lie after he already knew the game was up.

Some have suggested that Madoff might be a sociopath. After all, all sociopaths are narcissistic (though the reverse doesn't always follow). To me, there are details that lean towards NPD rather than ASPD. Despite his clear lack of remorse, he pleaded guilty to all 11 charges against him. This is not the behaviour of a sociopath. A sociopath would have played the game until the end, throwing others in front of the bus where necessary. He or she wouldn't care how their co-conspirators and victims perceived them.

Instead, Madoff's public admission of guilt serves two purposes. It makes him look honest and repentant to the general public. It also helps him to save face with his associates and co-conspirators. In fact, Madoff went as far as to reward loyal colleagues with generous gifts in the wake of his fall from grace. As if that could ever make up for the agonising pain he inflicted on these people and their families.

My sincere love and whole heart goes out to the souls of Ruth Madoff, Bernie's wife (who lost her husband and understanding of truth and life) and his two sons, Andrew (who died four years after his father's arrest as a result of cancer) and Mark (who sadly took his own life two years after his father's arrest). And, of course, to the many, many victims, directly and indirectly impacted by this man's disorder. Judge Denny Chin called the fraud 'extraordinarily evil' but Madoff will die arguing he is not evil, he is not a monster. At the time of writing this book, I personally added Bernie Madoff to Wikipedia's list of narcissists. It took great restraint not to add 'killer' to his list of occupations!

Jimmy Savile: the monster that fooled a nation

Where do we start with Jimmy Savile? In hindsight, the evidence for this vile child abuser having a wicked and dangerous personality disorder is clear. It is almost as if his death broke a strange spell that rendered sensible people incapable of seeing the hideous truth behind the glamour.

It is unsettling to realise that, in many ways, Savile played the narcissist's game and won. He went to his grave with an OBE as Sir James Wilson Vincent Savile; he was treasured, in life, as a generous philanthropist; he was adored, by many, as a charismatic eccentric and he was even buried in the gold coffin he requested.

He was untouchable and he knew it. He openly told people that he wasn't interested in charities and disliked children, yet he still managed to pull the wool over people's eyes. Public bodies such as the BBC refused to air any accusations against him despite a widespread understanding that he 'liked them young'.

There is a power in having no empathy and no remorse. Savile was once interviewed by psychiatrist Dr Anthony Clare on BBC Radio 4 and he described this power as 'ultimate freedom', saying that he was one of only a few people who could claim to have it.

As we all know now, he used his so-called 'clout' in the most depraved, reprehensible way. After his death, hundreds of allegations began to flood in. It is now estimated that Savile's victims, mainly children, numbered more than 300 over more than half a century of abuse.

An arch-manipulator, Savile used his 'generosity' and status to gain unfettered access to Stoke Mandeville Hospital where he abused dozens of children.

Why did Savile commit such heinous crimes? Whereas a healthy person will accept feelings of low self-esteem, fear, shame and anger, the narcissist cannot bear them as they threaten to crack the fake persona that they have built-up over their lifetime.

For Savile, in common with other abusive narcissists, there was a simple solution. Make other people take on those feelings. His abuse will have been a way of disowning and projecting those unbearable feelings onto his helpless victims. Let them feel afraid, ashamed, weak and angry.

It has been reported that once Savile committed an act of sexual abuse, he would then quickly lose interest in that person. He discarded his victims, many of them hospitalised children, without a second thought. It was always about him, him, him.

Was Savile a psychopath? Although he claimed to have no feelings, this could well be a tactic to deflect attention away from exploring his inner psyche (how horrific to have to look inside such a soul). He even admitted that a scandal would leave him 'covered in shame'. Psychopaths don't feel ashamed.

Savile's obsession with his public image and status, his recognition of shame, and the enjoyment he seemed to have in humiliating and hurting his victims, suggests a severe and malignant case of NPD.

Narcissism on the big and small screen
- American Psycho
- Basic Instinct
- Blue Jasmine
- Cruel Intentions
- Election
- Gone Girl
- Gone with the Wind
- Joker
- Scapegoat

- Snow White and the Huntsman
- Sunset Boulevard
- The Girl on the Train
- The Hustle
- The Wizard of Lies
- The Wolf of Wall Street
- To Die For

The Hustle: fact or fiction?
For all its fun and silliness, a dark undertone runs through the 2019 film *The Hustle* with its portrayal of cold, calculating emotional and financial abuse.

Anne Hathaway, in particular, gives us a convincing portrayal of a true narcissist. Her character, Josephine Chesterton, has none of the redeeming empathy that bring us closer to Penny Rust, Rebel Wilson's character. With Josephine, we have all the traits of the dyed-in-the-wool NPD:

- The relentless pursuit of material gain.
- The ability to turn on the tears convincingly to abuse the empathy of another person.
- A callous disregard of other people's feelings.
- A complete lack of remorse.

And while Rebel Wilson shows a more human motivation to her hustling (no spoilers–you'll have to watch the film!), Anne Hathaway does what she does, simply because she can.

All popular films hook into timeless mythological dramas that play themselves out in the deepest recesses of our mind. While we may dismiss Josephine as a caricature (and in a way, she is), a part of us knows and fears that abusers like her are out there laying traps for the unwary. If you have doubts about that, the next chapter could change your mind. This real-life case study of a cold, ruthless NPD was the most chilling I have ever encountered. As such, I have included it in all its raw, stark detail.

CHAPTER 6

BLACK WIDOW:
A SHORT STORY OF LETHAL NPD

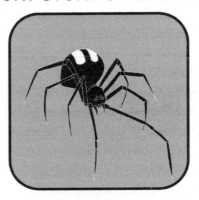

"O Rose thou art sick,
The invisible worm
That flies in the night
In the howling storm
Has found out thy bed
Of crimson joy
And his dark, secret love
Does thy life destroy."
-William Blake-

This chilling case of the Black Widow distils all aspects of my knowledge and experience of working with codependency and NPD into one chapter. It is deadly, true and oh-so-necessary. If I do nothing else in my life, I hope that this book warns people and saves them from their own personal hell. Yes, people often die at the hands of an NPD. It must stop. And in this strange world, where entitled people are being socially-produced more and more, I personally believe that evil NPDs are on the rise. This is a case that I am still working on, as this book goes to print. I am working with the legal teams and the victims. As such names, locations and other such details have been changed to protect the victims.

Robert's childhood

A boy was born to a couple who were very much in love. But things turned bad and went wrong very quickly. This vulnerable and fragile little baby started to feel hungry and scared. So early did this happen, that the boy never tasted the romantic sweetness that followed his parents' meeting, their wedding and, of course, the wonder of pregnancy.

Dad lost his job and got into the habit of heavy drinking, spending the little food and household money the family received on booze as soon as the government cheque came in. Robert's first years were spent living in a cold, damp cellar. The only light that came in was through a few tiny, slatted windows in the ceiling and these were always opaque with dust. It let Robert know whether it was day or night but provided no view to the outside world, no colour, no warmth.

At age five, having not moved from his squalid home and dire situation, Robert started school. He quickly understood that there was something special about his own situation.

He couldn't exactly put his finger on what this was but the other kids in his class seemed to have different stories to tell about their family pursuits and day-to-day lives. Fortunately, Robert was a bright kid and soon learned it was best to make up stories about his warm, soft and cuddly mummy and his fun dad whom he played with and who took him for ice-cream. He started to develop his imaginary world.

There were lots of arguments and fights. Sometimes, Mum would go quiet after a thump, a slap or often a throat-hold. It was the norm for Robert. He didn't know any different and yet he knew things needed to be different.

Robert became interested in books and comics about war, the military and self-defence. He had no money but he did have access to the local library and read extensively, as an escape. This was Robert's safe place, somewhere he always looked forward to going. The librarians and middle-aged clerks always behaved kindly towards him. They had warm smiles. Robert felt safe and warm in the library.

You may think that war and self-defence would be a strange interest for such a young boy. Not so if we consider that, aged seven, Robert's mother was beaten in front of him; the violence no longer contained behind the bedroom door. It got worse. Robert's father put a gun to his head and told him never to speak about what he saw or his head would be blown off. Things quietened at home when Robert's father found another woman to host his needs. Like a well-behaved narcissist, he left Robert and Mum in peace by finding another feeding ground elsewhere. He left without a flinch or a feeling.

For Robert and Mum, they had no money, little food and were living in the same cellar—but life was peaceful.

Robert's world changed on the day he peed himself while a gun was pointed at his head. Despite his tender age, he developed a life-saving vision. The vision was for his life to be better than this. He heard real stories at school about safe, warm and loving families. He wanted one of his own and visualised this; he was going to "make" this happen. He wasn't too sure how he would do it but he was certain he needed to get out of "this".

Without having any idea that he was suffering from PTSD at this vulnerable age, Robert's experiences affected his social skills and made him implode. At home, he tried to make his poor Mum happy and proud of him, but he lived in fear of not being able to defend her and himself. He was never going to feel weak and helpless again. He would never be bullied.

His new goal was to read more, and push himself more, to be the best in everything. He knew, without quite knowing why, that this was his ticket out of Dodge. He found that school was a consistent place for him to be rewarded and the more he worked, the better his grades were. He felt good about who he was in school and nurtured positive feelings about himself. He was consumed with happiness when he received affection from his teachers and the school environment, something he experienced nowhere else.

The making of Robert

Robert used his academic ability to realise his vision of being in the military and becoming like his self-defence heroes. By joining the military, he could finally escape from his cold, poor, depressed mother and his missing father.

He knew he couldn't accept being a gopher in the military; he needed to find a position of value. He became super fit, studied martial arts and developed an attitude to win and survive. He scored well in the military and was singled out to join a special forces division. This gave Robert huge confidence in his ability to turn his hopes into reality. The military, although strict, was his first real home. He was secure, had regular food, didn't have to worry about his mother and put every morsel of his soul into being a good soldier and comrade.

It was Robert's pure grit and fear that spurned him to the top, every time! Robert was also a keen people watcher. He studied the men he was serving with, people from all different financial backgrounds and class systems, and saw through to the real people within. He was becoming wiser and more capable every day.

After several years, Robert was offered an educational program to go into engineering. He focused on his studies and did extremely well, joining a university campus funded by the military. But once again, he felt the stark difference between the lives of the kids on campus and his own. Even though he was similar in age to his peers, he felt that he was the only kid with no family apart from his reliable military 'foster parents.'

He had nowhere to go on university break and received no care packages. However, he also realised that these kids, although mostly well to do, were less determined than him. They did not have as strong a vision as he did. They had very different motivations. Robert's motivation was to survive against all odds.

Very soon, during his time at university, Robert understood his vision needed updating and that a degree in engineering wouldn't be enough. If he was going to feel safe, loved and have a family, like the ones he'd heard about at school and university, Robert knew that he had to recreate himself again. His new vision was to become financially and romantically successful. But how?

The military were the parents Robert never had. These parents had taught him respect, order, ability, strength, self-belief, stamina, teamwork and obedience. However, above all, the military had taught Robert how to think outside of the box. It drummed into him how to develop new strategies, to question people's messages and words, and to always think three steps ahead of everyone else. All the while, he would be triple-checking that his own mind was clear while balancing caution with opportunity. Robert's natural strength was to be as sharp as a tack. Even as a young child he was very aware of his surroundings and he could process the world very quickly.

Robert, having completed university and worked his time out of the military, joined a new-fangled software company against the advice of a few of his friends and mentors. Unlike them, he could see that the world was changing; he could see what products people would need and what processes might help them.

Robert felt deep in his stomach, as he had about joining the military, that this was his ticket to family and security. He worked 16 hours a day, left no stone unturned and pushed forward with military determination to succeed, which he did. He developed software that truly worked and he realised that his ideas and developments were indeed very much needed.

The power of Robert's motivation was pushing him to levels of strategy and ability that surpassed anything he could have imagined. This was scary but exciting. At times, he believed in himself but then he would be racked with insecurity.

He found he could think smarter than most of his peers, as he was more attuned to the target than to his colleagues' personal egos. He took care of the job at hand and refused to allow emotions or personal struggles to have an impact on him. But beneath it all, Robert's main terror simmered away. A fear of not being loved, of being unlovable, of never finding a family of his own and, worst of all, of having to go back to his previous life underneath the street. This made Robert unstoppable and his success sometimes shocked him. He found that money talked. A nice suit, tie and shirt talked. He would often do a double take when eating out at the restaurants he had once walked past and thought were out of his reach. Even now, Robert takes a second glance and wonders if this is all real.

Love and family

Finally, romance came in the form of a PA he met at a bar. She worked for one of the companies he was working with. They were in love (Robert was not certain of what that was but he found this woman attractive and fun and they shared some similar likes). It was not long before they were married but Robert continued working long hours and they had to move countries several times. He finally took the plunge and started working on his own projects.

During this time, his wife fell pregnant with their first child, which spurred Robert on even more to fight to the finish line. He put his products on the market and started to make money. Enough to provide a house, food and a good environment for his family.

He continued working crazy hours and the couple had two more children whom he adored. The more he adored them, the more he put his foot on the accelerator to make absolutely certain they would never live in the cellar of his nightmares. Robert continued striving until one day he sold his small company for unimaginable amounts of money. His financial vision was becoming real.

As part of the sale agreement, for several years Robert was forbidden from working for another company and from promoting himself. For tax reasons, he was also advised to move to the Cayman Islands and wait out his time there until he could work or develop products again. This did not go too well for his family or him. He had tunnel vision and was not sure how to manage this very wealthy life.

He turned his attention to the stock market, learning how to invest and make his money work for him. This was a whole new world to Robert and it soon became apparent that the pressure of sudden wealth, moving the whole family to a different country and having the military as a parenting template were not sustainable. Robert loved being an at-home dad but his wife was missing her country, home, family and friends. Unfortunately, the marriage became cold and unloving.

Robert also found himself in an impossible situation with his sons. They had grown up in private schools within the kind of privileged circumstances that he had always vowed to provide for them. But, unlike Robert, his boys had been encouraged to express themselves and question the world. They were not obedient to military standards. In the military a person never answered back! When you were told you had to do something, you did it out of respect and because you knew it was for the common good. Robert, who knew no different, found he had to put his boys in line at times, as they seemed ungrateful and disrespectful.

He constantly overcompensated for his own deplorable

childhood. Despite his best intentions, Robert started to drink quite heavily and his anger and military method of control would cause severe tension in his family unit. Needless to say, the long-term marriage did not last much longer and an ugly separation ensued. Robert lost the ideal family he had striven so hard to build. As a result of his sadness and depression, his finances suffered too. Robert nose-dived into despair. Time passed and the contractual restrictions of not competing in the world of software lifted. Robert started to look to invest in companies.

At the time of the divorce, Robert, who is very kind, responsible and generous, agreed to pay his ex-wife US$13 million cash together with an equally generous package to take care of his sons, which included sending them to top schools and universities. There was never a doubt that Robert would stand by his parental obligations. Having been abandoned by a father who never took an interest in him and broke promises, Robert made a pledge to his sons. He would do the right thing by them.

Still, his bitter and vindictive ex-wife wanted more money, so she hit him with a US$110 million lawsuit. After they had separated, Robert cleaned up his act, he stopped drinking and feeling sorry for himself. He directed this energy into his career once more and made some healthy decisions that brought in several hundred million dollars. His wife filed for half of it even though she had already signed all the contracts and had not contributed to the new earnings. She was also the one who had withheld sex for 10 years, had failed to support Robert in his struggles and had focused on turning the children against him. In fact, she was the one who had really pushed for the divorce in the first place, yet seemed vindictive and angry when Robert agreed and moved on with his life.

Robert lost all respect for her when she used the children as her weapons against him. For the past two years (at the time of writing this) Robert's sons have not seen their father. Their mother is using every tactic in the book to keep them from him, twisting truths and provoking guilt when they show him affection.

Robert spent millions to defend this long, drawn out and exhausting divorce. He was again left without a family and with his dreams in the gutter. He had no idea why his boys were not good soldiers and how his marriage had grown so cold. The divorce took eight years to finalise, eight years of a battle that has harmed his relationship with his boys. And for what?

He successfully developed products again, even more of them than before. He invested in new innovations. Over the next decade, he was growing in business but his relationship with his estranged wife was still difficult and this was further spilling over into his relationship with the boys whom she continued to poison against him. Although Robert still maintains a relationship with them, he's realising, through our therapeutic work, that his military parenting really didn't serve him well in all aspects of being a father. He didn't beat his children (although he occasionally clipped their ears) but he was severe on his boundaries and struggled to understand that they were from a different world to him.

Now he wishes he'd known better. He doesn't understand what it is like for children to go through a privileged education and be well-to-do university students, to be brought up as multi-millionaires, living in the nicest houses, attending the best parties and receiving the highest quality possessions. Parenting can be a thankless task at the best of times but worse when the parents are at war.

He did his best for his sons at the time but his father had been terribly brutish and his mother had been non-existent, so he had no benchmark. But he is learning how to parent and is bridging a relationship with his children. They are mostly unresponsive at the time of writing this but they are smart and with time and thought they may see a future.

He is becoming more understanding that his sons have their own minds and their own ways of doing things, and that that is "okay".

After getting back on his feet, Robert dated a few girls but said he wasn't interested in spending time with someone who looked absolutely brilliant but had no brains. He found one night stands unfulfilling; in fact, after sex they left him feeling empty.

He was really looking for a partner in life, a warmth he desired but as yet had never found. Finally, in 2015, he went to an elite dating agency as suggested by a friend.

Enter the Black Widow
Even with all his military training, intellect, stamina and strength, Robert could never have prepared himself for what was to happen next. So, there he is, broken-hearted but with all the money in the world, when along comes RR. To Robert, she seemed smart, switched on and beautiful although, in hindsight, she didn't feel quite right. However, most irresistible of all, she seemed to quickly fall deeply in love with him. Robert was being introduced to many contenders by the agency but

RR persisted most, chased him even. Of course, that's the first thing a narcissist does! They put you on a pedestal, make you out to be the best thing in the world and then boom! The games start.

Let's be mindful here. Robert didn't know she was married at first nor that she had bought a house with her husband just four months earlier. Why would he when the agency promotes the serious vetting of its members, both male and female? Robert understood anyone being promoted to him had to have a clean "bill of health": independently wealthy and safe to be introduced to.

When RR revealed her history, she convinced Robert she was divorcing her husband—but she wasn't—she didn't even start divorcing him until three years later. What she did do immediately was to start negotiating a way forward with Robert—and that involved tens of thousands of dollars in regular payments and then millions of dollars upfront. She would tell him that was the cost of 'exclusivity'. "If you want to marry me, I need millions, I need security, I have a child." Robert was no match for this street girl who adored nice handbags.

The first six months, in Robert's words, "progressed slowly". The pair spent some time together on Robert's boat but didn't have sex until 2016 (a control feature that was to become worse and worse). Robert accepted that this was the pace RR wanted to go at. He was attracted to her and was excited by the hope of a blossoming relationship.

As time went on, RR learnt what Robert liked sexually and carried out the research necessary to reel him in; Robert described sex as "the strongest glue" between them. He also went along with her wishes to keep the relationship low profile. She would only really date Robert in inconspicuous venues and would never allow public displays of affection in her home town. She never introduced him to her close friends and family and didn't tell them about her and Robert's future plans. He did not exist in her world. Did she have a world?

And then, in the summer of 2016, RR declared she wanted another child, which made Robert leap with joy. Robert, understandably, demanded that she must now divorce her husband and move in with him before becoming pregnant.

But even while Robert was pursuing this relationship, RR was busy building her network of wealthy contacts.

For example, in 2017, RR and Robert were at a prestigious corporate event when she began to give out her personal business cards rather than their joint ones. This angered Robert and they quarrelled. On reflection, Robert recognises that she was on an NPD "fishing expedition", looking for the next big catch. Just like Bernie Madoff, she was interested only in building relationships with high net worth individuals who could sustain a lifestyle she saw herself as entitled to. This is a person that has never really worked a day in her life to contribute—bar having sex with people for compensation. Not as a healthy sex worker with boundaries but as a scammer.

She wasn't interested in what was in their hearts—just what was in their bank accounts!

In November of that year, RR announced that she was pregnant. At first she said the child was Robert's but then she revealed it was her husband's child. At the time, Robert couldn't fathom what was real and what wasn't. RR quickly flashed Robert a document from an IVF clinic explaining that this was how she had become pregnant: with her husband's sperm and her egg. Robert admits he didn't study the document closely. He was in shock. His world fell apart again. He was heartbroken, struggling for reason and, as all good codependents do, he kept looking for some idea of what he had done wrong to deserve this. He did leave her; he broke off the relationship for a couple of months, but even though her explanation was so unbelievable, Robert successful—a kind, honest, intelligent and thoughtful (but not streetwise) person—learned to accept it. Robert's internal dialogue was like a hamster wheel:

"Oh yes, of course she wants another baby because she has always wanted two children. And she did use IVF! Why didn't she want my child? Well, naturally she wanted the two children to have the same father. . ."

And Robert kept on reasoning and reasoning and reasoning and reasoning because this is what gaslighting is used for. It makes us start to try and find some reason in the chaos whilst repeating, "I don't understand!" He was continually told that "he" was unreasonable and that "he" was ruining everything.

He accepted it all because he was living in hope that this beautiful, smart woman, the one who had given him the best six months of his life, truly wanted him and was going to build a life with him. He stayed hooked because, in his words, "She knows how to put on a show. She knows how to perform in order to keep the victim, like myself, hanging there."

Once RR learned about Robert's troubled childhood, she added that knowledge to her NPD arsenal. By mimicking Robert's own story, she knew she could trigger his empathy. He would forgive RR's bad behaviours because he could relate to her pain—but was that a complete charade too? Robert was trying to heal his own past by healing RR's but somehow it didn't work, Robert kept failing and she kept reminding him of that.

They were soon back together again and the negotiations over money continued. RR would use Robert's insecurities against him, warning him that if he didn't give her the security she needed, someone else would appreciate her qualities. These she would then reel off (she was beautiful, glamorous, a real lady, interesting, smart, caring, sporty, young, good-looking, etc). She would say that Robert might have his millions but he would inevitably become an alcoholic and lose his kids. With all of this, she was threatening to take away the three things he desired most in life: to be safe, to be loved and to be wanted.

Just after the baby was born, Robert and RR came to me. I very quickly realised the situation that Robert was in and while I refused to work with them as a couple, I gladly took on Robert's case. RR spent the whole intake session telling me that I had to diagnose Robert with NPD, that it is clear he is mean, that he tells lies all the time, that he abuses her with power and promises he does not keep. All her own issues being projected upon Robert. How did I make such a quick determination? Codependents always search themselves for reason and everything being their fault. NPDs immediately blame everything on everyone else with remorse being absent. She fitted the mould. And, this is where I entered this battle.

As I explained earlier in this book, many narcissists bolster their egos with material possessions and will go to elaborate lengths in order to support their sense of superiority and their fantasies. And so it was with RR. Whenever they visited somewhere, she would go out shopping and spend US$30,000 on handbags, and US$20,000 on shoes, or have couturier fashion companies come to the hotel and choose her a dress for the evening. But Robert loved and adored her. He thought, 'This must be the one after all my turmoil, all the fighting in court, all the bimbos and the bars. This must be the one'. Although Robert loved her, he was the unhappiest he had ever been in his life. Like a cocaine user, the highs when he got the fix were great but all the down times, irritability and vast confusion that went with this were certainly not peaceful. Little did he know that she was buying things to turn into cash later. Her husband had lost his job for insider trading and they needed money: Robert's money.

And like Anne Hathaway in the movie The Hustle, she was the best damned actress. She could make herself cry on demand. I have seen video footage of her negotiating and whenever her argument was exposed as weak, she would cry and then project everything "she was" on to Robert saying that he was selfish, he was narcissistic, he did whatever he pleased, he was violent, he was brutal and so on. But he wasn't. It was all her. They broke up but soon got back together again.

Secrets and surveillance

In 2018, when Robert's son wanted some one-on-one time with his dad on his yacht, RR took the private jet back to their family home in Chicago with the two children and two nannies (at home she has three nannies, but she only travelled with two!).

Robert's son had a minor accident and had to return home and cancel his trip with dad. So Robert invited RR back to the boat, suggesting they took a holiday trip.

RR exploded, screaming, "No! You can't just ask me to change plans like that. Who the f*** do you think you are? I've got to go to this 70th birthday party in San Francisco. You're disgusting Robert! What's wrong with you? You don't own me. I have my own friends, I have my own life, I have my own people." Robert had just given her US$300,000 as she promised she was going to sign the cohabitation agreement and move in with him. They had only been spending around 40 days each year together.

More gaslighting.

She was actually going to be with her secret lover, a well-known, well-connected, almost billionaire businessman (VV) whom she was seeing behind Robert's back. Clearly, RR had her focus further up the food chain but who is predator and who is prey in this new deadly dance? I find it interesting that VV refers to himself as American Royalty.

What RR didn't realise was that Robert had been tipped off, so he had surveillance follow her. When she was spotted with the man in a restaurant, Robert decided again he'd had enough and couldn't take the pain, confusion, hurt and loneliness (abuse) anymore.

He got surveillance to pass her a note saying, 'Hello Little Princess, it's over. I'm gone!'

The note was delivered to her in front of VV during an intimate dinner at one of the best restaurants in Los Angeles (honeymoon phase?). Robert felt good, then terrible, then started to doubt himself again. RR had his mind so twisted that he felt that without her he would be nothing. His mind was reeling. Did this mean that everything was his fault and he was bad. Did RR being with VV prove her point? Had he been thinking wrong all this time? He did not know what was sensible and what was fake anymore. He was completely off anchor. He had just agreed with her that she was going to marry him. He had plummeted from ecstatic to horrified and desperately sad.

Some days later, RR retaliated with a stream of aggression and crazy excuses. She said, "I was at a birthday. I was just in town and happened upon him. You always make me out to be bad. You always say I'm telling you lies. You always try to control me. You just have to f*** off. You don't know anything that's happening in my f****** life". Note that narcissists create fantasies which then become their worlds. They believe everything they say and do, so their lies are naturally very convincing to the outside world. In true Eliza Doolittle form, when cornered, RR would revert to true form, with a potty mouth and vile abuse.

This time though, Robert couldn't believe her wild, forceful explanations. After all, he now had video evidence of her using the keypad to VV's mansion and letting herself in. She had spent time overnight with him, several times, over this period. Robert was living his own feared hell. He felt unloved, abandoned and discarded. His world had fallen away from him. He had no certainty under his feet. He was desperate beyond belief. During this brutal time, we very nearly lost Robert. I had to tell him that this would be very unfair to himself and his boys. We kept Robert safe with regular sessions and agreements. It was a very, very dark time.

Once again Robert and RR broke up; this time for several months.

However, as we found out recently, VV was not about to

put a ring on RR's finger or give her an immediate share of his money. He clearly isn't as adept at playing the codependent role. Maybe RR was realising that she could be in for a battle trying to land this shark because, in true NPD style, she started to hedge her bets by calling Robert again, assuring him that the affair was over and that they had a beautiful future together, showing him photographs of how good they looked together.

RR convinced Robert to put a quarter of a million dollars in her bank account immediately. This was on the promise that she loved him truly and that she would sign a cohabitation contract with him. US$2.5 million and US$50,000 of a US$5 million and US$50,000 payment was to be secured in a Cayman Islands bank account at the beginning of the signing of the contracts, which happened in December 2019. The remaining US$2.5 million was to be put in escrow until they got married (which was planned for September 2020). In truth, it was a very one-sided agreement which even stated that should Robert break the cohabitation agreement, she would still get all the money! It surprises me that Robert's lawyers ever sanctioned his signing of such a document. The legal team I am working with alongside Robert state the same. Robert was taken for a ride.

RR and Robert got engaged for the second time in December 2019, in Paris. It was a well-planned and elaborate engagement, executed lovingly by Robert; he was excited because he believed all the horrors were now past them and a wonderful future lay ahead. Maybe, just maybe, something had changed. I, in true therapeutic style, went along with this and worked with Robert's happy times. However, I felt very nervous and filled with rage at how this was unfolding. I took this rage to clinical supervision and we reasoned that this was not my stuff but part of the transference of this very trying case.

It was proven shortly afterwards that RR was continuing to see VV over that period. What was he promising her? Were they hatching plots together? Was RR still running the show or was VV now pulling the strings, his greedy eyes on Robert's wealth?

Robert became suspicious when she would not join him in the Cayman Islands as COVID-19 developed. In fact, she kept as far from him as possible after their engagement except during a short trip to Mexico and a week's stay on his yacht. Even then, she was not engaging in sex. Robert felt <u>she</u> needed time to heal.

The alarm bells really started ringing again when she kept putting off moving in with him until January 31 2021. She mistakenly thought that cohabitation was automatically confirmed then but the document clearly stated that the agreement was secure and valid only if she and Robert were in an 'enduring and loving relationship' by that date.

Things developed further. When the COVID-19 lockdown ended, Robert travelled to Chicago and discovered that all RR had moved in to their future home were a few personal items; it was like she had been staying at an Airbnb. Nor did she welcome him as a lover that she had not seen for weeks and weeks. Instead, she disappeared several times each day and spent one whole day, 14 hours, at her ex-husband's home nearby. Be mindful, she does not work, has three nannies and a housekeeper, yet is always too busy to invest in Robert. To the point of being ridiculously aloof and precious.

Robert again ordered surveillance on RR to assist in evidencing (or disproving) that this was a con. Robert's home is a multi-million dollar mansion and nearby, there's a private garden that she kept visiting to have phone conversations.

She continued to spend most of her time at her ex-husband's home and was filmed having conversations as she walked through the nearby parks and streets. Surveillance found out that her conversation partners included VV and a therapist. RR goes through such people: nannies, housekeepers, lawyers and therapists, quickly. This was thought to be another new therapist.

The next time Robert flew in from the Cayman Islands, RR again spent all day and night at her ex-husband's house. This time, she told him that it was because she had to write a 30-page child protection document against her ex-husband. That was the exact moment Robert decided to have her followed by his security officers. Her ex-husband was talking to Robert's legal team so something did not sit right. Using FaceTime, they recorded her and could hear and see everything she was saying. It turned out that she was still having conversations with VV, sometimes several times each day. The surveillance team threw microphones into the gardens next to her and recorded her having a conversation with her 'therapist'. She was explaining to them that everything was fake with Robert and that it was all about her future security and the money.

For Robert, it was the moment that broke through all of his illusions. He heard her tell her therapist that she felt her heart was with VV, that they were soul mates, and that she had never loved Robert. She admitted she couldn't even touch Robert and that it had all been for security.

Robert felt he could easily chalk off the US$5 million, not

a problem, but he couldn't accept how he had been taken in and made out to be a fool; how he had been deceived into entering into a legal agreement with RR; how he was the last to know what was really going on.

All this time, he had thought he was sharing his most intimate moments with RR but it had all been part of her working financial plan. He had been an expendable piece of her life, someone who had been of service to her but in whom she was incapable of being interested.

What also plays on Robert's mind is that she doesn't even take care of her own children, an issue that is close to his heart because Robert feels strongly about the welfare of all children. He had spent five years of his life getting to know RR's children and had hoped he could help to support and love them in the future too. He had spent time and money designing and furnishing the children's rooms in the house they were supposed to have shared, twice! RR never took an interest and Robert even pays for her three nannies. RR spends very little time with her children. When she does, it's for little more than to take selfies for social media or to use as another strong hook to keep Robert in her grips. She's reporting that she's fighting her husband for custody and Robert fears for their futures. Growing up with a narcissistic mother will be disastrous for them.

Robert has good people in his world. For example, he has a CEO in charge of the family business, a super smart businessman who supports him in any business dealings. In fact, just 18 months ago, a convincing bogus company wanted over US$100 million in investment from them but when they did their checks, following five months of around the world negotiations, they realised the company didn't have the substance to back them up, so they pulled out.

So, how could Robert and his protectors spot and avoid a clever business scam yet remain blind to RR's deception? First, Robert was so afraid of being alone and unloved that he preferred to cling to the illusion of love and future happiness rather than examine the facts with his usual cold eye of logic. Second, Robert's protectors didn't intervene, despite their misgivings, because they respected that this was Robert's personal life.

RR was—and continues to be—a financial and emotional parasite without remorse. She is at the same level as a paedophile. She will coach someone who is vulnerable, make them feel special and then use them for her own needs and gratification. All the while, in true NPD fashion, she claims, and above all believes, that it was all Robert, the victim's problem. Robert wanted this and thus he had brought it upon himself. Zero remorse and zero learning.

But despite all of her scheming, planning and cold advantage, she messed up. She messed up because she didn't realise that in the middle of a private garden, microphones could be thrown next to her and she could be listened to. She could be followed and filmed whilst on FaceTime. Her usual crooked and scheming way of being did not go undetected. Most people just cannot believe the audacity of such people and this is the one reason why they get away with so much. Their pure, unreproached audacity.

Of course, not everyone has the resources or connections to discover this type of demon in action. However, it is hoped most sincerely that you understand that Robert, with all his history of abuse, training and support team, would have probably married RR and even wound up mysteriously dead if he had not witnessed the unbelievable evidence for himself. The mean trick of the NPD is to rely upon the hopes and fears of their prey.

What can we learn from this? If it seems too good to be true, it probably is. If it seems too unreasonable to be reasonable, it probably is. Healthy and kind people do not understand such audacity and cruelty.

A kind, thoughtful person with integrity who can love and wants to be loved will always have some self-doubt. Couple this with a childhood of abuse and no support or healthy example of family life and boom! To the NPD, this is the scent of a perfect host and they will sniff it out.

Has RR also messed up in another way? Has she bitten off more than she can chew with VV? The more he has become involved in the story, the more I ponder whether he has an agenda of his own—and how far he is prepared to go to push it.

The net closes

Codependents often live in dire fear of what could happen. Even with his own military precision and the support of top international lawyers and myself, Robert harboured self-doubts in the 24 hours leading up to the envelope being delivered to RR. This envelope contained documents stating that the game was up. And most importantly, and sadly, for Robert, the engagement was also off; in fact, it was never real and neither was the cohabitation agreement. The one thing this letter did not state was that she was to stop cohabitating (that would have triggered a clause in the agreement leading to Robert losing his US$5 million-plus).

All the night before RR was served the documents, Robert tossed and turned, went over all the information again, considered what he was doing and felt nauseous, scared of what retaliation there might be. He sent messages to the lawyers and me several times. He was living his darkest fear. He had made himself vulnerable and faced the ultimate in humiliation and loneliness. We had many sessions through this time to hold Robert to sift through the what-ifs, grief and sickened realities.

Meanwhile, surveillance video and audio footage continued to come in. RR clearly knew something was up. She had been followed for weeks now and her behaviour was changing. She could be seen darting in and out of doorways with her hood up and an umbrella (even when it wasn't raining). She would walk the streets for two to three hours at a time talking to people on FaceTime. Whenever she stopped, she learned to put her back to the railings or wall so that nobody could look over her shoulder.

Then all of a sudden, the day before the 'sting operation' in May 2020, when the team felt they had sufficient evidence, RR conveniently sat on a bench, within audio recording range, and had a frank discussion with what seemed to be another new therapist. She was talking to them as if guiding them to help her in a child custody and car ownership case with her husband. She also spoke about how her appalling childhood had led her to be who she is today and how that was probably driving her to make bad decisions. The leading lawyer and I both thought it seemed staged, too convenient.

The meeting between Robert, the lawyers and myself was

calm. They asked for me to define NPD a little better for them so they understood what they were going to be dealing with. Just 15 minutes before we were going to be in the meeting, the sting operation took place and the surveillance team took the legal firm's process server to deliver the letter to RR. As soon as she had it in her hand, she was sent an email and, in accordance with the law, her lawyer was also sent an email.

We had many conversations between Robert, the lawyers and myself.

I needed to make it clear that my part in these meetings was to help Robert be safe, monitor his risk situation and have him feel supported (and also to keep Robert safe from himself and RR). The lawyers agreed that if Robert instigated any communication whatsoever between himself and RR it could jeopardise the contractual case and Robert's safety. It was agreed that Robert would block all his devices, social media, email, WhatsApp and text and would have no communication with RR for the next five days. The lead lawyer and myself made ourselves available for this period should Robert need our support. The pain we witnessed in Robert was severe and unsettling. I doubled my own clinical supervision so that I could be supported and also to double check my work. This period was so dark I needed to check in and revisit my part and role in this.

RR and her ex-husband's home remained under 24-hour surveillance and the reports went to the lead lawyer so that if anything untoward happened, he could involve us. In that way, Robert would be shielded from being constantly reminded of every treacherous step RR was taking.

But Robert was unable to be so passive. He felt he should

draw on his military training and take part in the surveillance. This did enable him to contribute significantly by observing her actions after being served. It also, unexpectedly, helped with some healing by taking away his remaining doubts about RR. She was cold, calculated and almost indifferent throughout the entire process. 24 hours of observational evidence tells us much about a person!

This case has truly left me with a haunting, stomach-churning sickness. Every kind, reasonable, thoughtful person wants to be wrong when they think of somebody as being capable of this level of abhorrence and selfishness.

It transpired that RR was using a barrister and lawyers and spending umpteen thousands of dollars to fight her ex-husband over the US$16,000 family car. One of the recorded phone calls picked up on her demanding Robert lie to lawyers and to the court about selling his US$140,000 vehicle. Robert was heard saying, "No, I am not going to lie for you. I am sick of hearing about your ex-husband" but she kept on insisting, "You will do this for me. Robert, I need you to say you're selling the car so that I don't have one and can tell the court that I need the family car and he can't have it." On the back of that, she was also rushing Robert for a payment of US$89,000 for the nannies—without even supplying an invoice! Her ex-husband had already been drained and ripped off by RR but she clearly wanted everything from him. She wouldn't stop taking until she was done and he was empty.

And these are RR's morals. A person who received over quarter of a million dollars in cash, has five and a half million dollars in Cayman Islands accounts and has also been given over a million dollars' worth of cash, gifts and jewellery—all under a fake guise of being in love with Robert and wanting to marry him and spend and share the rest of her life with him. But this NPD also wants her ex-husband's second hand, US$16,000 car. Where's the sense?

A twist soon came to this case when we wondered how and by whom intimate working pictures of RR were being taken. They were always taken at her marital home and in positions and places where she would need another person's help to take them. Also, it was revealed that her husband was fired from his job for illegal activity and that they needed money. Then, it became clear that her husband's new job just could not supply the enormous amount of money he was paying her: US$100,000 plus mortgage payment plus his rental (as he had left the marital home. None of this made sense and he refused to give a statement despite having called Robert's lawyers many times to give information about his children and then ex-wife. RR used a communication she found on her ex-husband's phone regarding a night out involving cocaine as a final ploy to get full custody of the children. She omitted (and he never challenged) the fact that she herself had a long and extensive history of drug use, including cocaine. She and her ex-husband also had a huge quantity of packages delivered to their home and Robert's home. In addition, there is a friendly and oft-talked about connection between RR and a famous cartel in Mexico. There is also, of course, VV somewhere in the mix. We know no more than this.

More games and gaslighting

This is a pure case of delusional and lethal NPD. And it feels strange to sit here and reflect and write about it. I feel we're in this space where Robert has legal support, emotional support, bodyguards and security agents looking after him. Still, I fear that if there's a tiny crack somewhere and if she can get one tiny fingernail through it to hook him, Robert will be back to where he was. This really feels unreal writing this. It is unreal! Unfathomable! It is absurd. This strong, intelligent, kind, wealthy man has almost been annihilated three times. In the last five years, since meeting RR, she has had a baby with her husband and didn't divorce him for three years, yet she still has a way of hooking Robert in, blaming him and projecting on to him everything that's bad about her. Engaged twice! Unimaginable.

Every healthy parent questions whether they are a good enough mum or dad or not and RR uses this against Robert. She has been saying, "You're a disgusting father to your three sons. No wonder they don't want to have anything to do with you," using every lethal, hateful, criminal way of getting his heart in her hands and squeezing it.

For Robert's sake and for the sake of any future vulnerable, kind and thoughtful person, I hope she's stopped now, forever. I always feel for the people I support in my work. This case has got under my skin too. Despite the extra supervision, it has left me with troubled nights and a sense of deep despair. Driving to Walmart a few months ago, I had an urgent message to call Robert. From the parking lot of Walmart I was presented with the task of talking Robert away from a cliff edge in the pouring rain, crying about RR's poor children and how he cannot take the pain anymore. We talked for over an hour. We helped Robert get to safety and understand he needed to be safe. I checked in with the lawyers about the concerns regarding the children and their safety. The lawyers explained that there were no grounds for a case of child abuse, nothing we could do. It pained my soul as I have always made it my mission to give children a voice and I was powerless. Shortly after this episode, RR took both children to Mexico for a month. Mexico at that time was one of the worst COVID-hit countries. She travelled alone and had the children follow with their nannies. Nothing more to say. Bless them.

With new evidence continuing to mount against RR, Robert will more than likely win his case. She has clearly breached most conditions of their contract and proven, without doubt that she was 'working' Robert, which is good from a legal perspective.

For the first time ever working on an NPD case, I was privileged to view 48 hours' worth of surveillance footage post the serving of the documents. Nothing much happened on the day RR was served but on the following day, all of a sudden, a removal truck turned up. Now, the legal documents she was served pointed out several break clauses which applied to her contract with Robert. One of these would apply if she hadn't actually moved in with him. In typical NPD-style again, she organised this large removal truck to come to Robert's property and within five hours, she had 'moved out' and taken her belongings 'back' to her ex-husband's house along with many of Roberts belongings. However, she was putting on a show. You could see that almost all of the boxes were either empty or contained one piece of clothing each. The removal people were almost carrying them with one finger on each box. They must have wondered what was going on but clearly, she had said she needed 100 or so boxes to make it look like she had just moved a whole truckload of possessions.

She even totally emptied the fridge, the freezer and the liquor and pantry cupboards. I guess she needed to put something into the boxes! So, this is her both gaslighting Robert and, once again, staging a fake scenario. She is more than likely planning to use the record from the moving company as proof of her sincerity. That record will prove the moving company packed 100 boxes although she is well aware that it won't prove what was—or was not—in the boxes.

More interesting footage was to come. The first person she contacted was her ex-husband and he arrives at the house to pick her up in his US$16,000 car, the one she is adamant about possessing. He then drives her around the corner (of course the surveillance team are following) and he starts banging the dash and screaming at her. RR starts to cry and he drives her back around the corner to Robert's house. She can clearly turn the tears on or off at the blink of an eye and they certainly seemed to stop her ex-husband from shouting. Other surveillance clocked him spending extended periods of time in Robert's house and the pair having a picnic together. This seems at odds with the supposed legal battles they are undergoing. Is that more deceit? More gaslighting? I don't understand, I just don't understand.

The next thing RR does, the day of the sting operation, is to go into the local grocery store and buy two SIM cards. At this point she is cold, like a reptile. She isn't acting at all like the love of her life, her future husband, has just said, "The deal's off. We understand what's really been going on." She is devoid of emotion.

We all, as humans, have doubt at times so it wasn't until that point, when I saw for myself the surveillance footage of her buying those two SIM cards, that I was 110% sure of my call on her being an NPD. To her, Robert wasn't a human being she had been messing with, and occasionally intimate with, for all those years. She had no regard for him at all. She seemed to have no regard for her children. She had no regard for anyone. VV? Is he next? Or is he now calling the shots? Has RR finally met her match? If so, a power battle between two narcissists would not be for the faint-hearted. It would be a fight to the death (or to the ruin of the loser).

As I watched the videos of RR's activities, it was like looking at a cold, soulless machine. And as I was feeling that, I looked down further through the surveillance footage and saw that the head of the surveillance team, a renowned ex-military special agent, was saying that she was a pro. He had no doubt about it: she had done this before. She knew exactly what she was doing. A cold mother, a machine, a robot. A drug dealer? A killer?

RR had been given four days to respond to Robert's lawyer's communication. Robert stated categorically that there was only one response he wanted to hear to avoid arbitration and that was, "I'm returning all the jewellery and gifts (worth one and a half million), cash (worth a million) and US$5,050,000 from the accounts." Instead, RR's lawyers came back with a brand-new accusation of harassment and a threat to report him to the police. There was no denial of the accusations against her—just more gaslighting designed to rattle Robert and presumably provoke him into making a fatal mistake.

Robert was now prepared to raise the stakes and enter into a very expensive and time-consuming arbitration. By trying to rake up dirt on Robert, RR was continuing her twisted game but to honest Robert, this was painfully real. She had crossed a boundary and he made it clear that he was now prepared to win at all costs. He doesn't want to destroy RR but he now demanded justice.

RR and her lawyers may yet come up with more legal tactics (after all, she has 24 hours a day to work on the case). However, Robert's legal team are ready for the fight.

Robert also wants to stop her doing this to anyone else. He's beyond being embarrassed about what he calls his "stupidity" and he understands that it's a strength to help prevent others from experiencing the same trauma. One of the most interesting things that Robert said to me in a recent session was that he had seen me use the DSM-5 as part of the legal process and he had had no prior idea that these mental health situations existed. He realised he had been a victim of five years of cold, hurtful, damaging, lethal abuse and wanted to know why people weren't taught about this. He was insistent about how we needed to get this message out to people, to prevent people from all walks of life becoming victims of people like RR. Hence the concept for this chapter was born.

Robert has been left in a very vulnerable position. Despite being a very successful and very intelligent person, he has had to trust in legal procedures in order to be protected.

Only when he feels that the legal case is being managed well enough can we think about his next steps towards healing. The most difficult thing for him is not knowing what was real and what wasn't. . . and if it were all fake, all just a con, where does this leave him? Or were parts of it real and special? Cries of, "I don't understand, I don't understand," echo in the corridors of Robert's mind in RR's wake. He doesn't know where he is.

I explained the grieving process to Robert and told him

that J. William Worden, one of the world's most renowned bereavement scholars, said, "Sometimes successful grieving is learning to live without the answers." This is especially true in very complicated grief cases.

I also explained to Robert that he needs to consider not undermining the extent, severity and longevity of the abuse he has experienced from RR. He needs to allow himself time to heal.

And it is abuse. The abuse of someone's kind nature. The abuse of their desire to help. The abuse of their empathy. The ruthless drive to get into a codependent's soul and have no regards, no respect, no morals. Just to keep on plugging away until they have taken everything from their host, everything!

I've seen so much destruction over my quarter of a century career working with victims of NPDs. I've even seen codependents in a much worse position than Robert.

I've seen victims who worked their whole life for a deposit on a property, met an NPD and ended up without the NPD and without two pennies to rub together, feeling worthless and heartbroken. After bleeding them dry, the narcissist leaves, without remorse, to find the next host and to get what they need to keep fulfil their next fantasy. Of course, it's always everybody else's fault, never theirs.

I have worked with people who have tried to kill themselves and haven't succeeded but have ended up with horrific injuries. I had a patient in a wheelchair who had jumped from the fifth storey of a building because she had been in a relationship with an NPD. She had signed over property and had nothing left. But she survived the jump and is now paralysed from the waist down. Some I've lost because they did manage to complete suicide. There are many cases where I don't even know what happened to the codependent because they returned to the NPD and never returned to me. It is my sincerest hope that someday the law criminalises NPDs for their actions and regards NPD as part of severe domestic violence. They are silent killers operating under the radar.

Be aware: a narcissist doesn't even have to be a super smart or insightful person, just plain ruthless, creating chaos and harm with their focused, lethal actions, all carried out without feeling.

Our disbelief and attempt to apply our own kind, smart reasoning to their aberrant behaviour is what they rely upon. One of the first things I do in therapy is to separate out the codependent and get them out of their abuser's head.

If a person maintains strict boundaries and is assertive, the parasite will move on swiftly to someone who is vulnerable. Otherwise, they would be unable to feed adequately and keep their fantasy world going.

At times, Robert spoke about society being broken and there being no truth in the world. He can't understand how RR can sign a cohabitation deal all the while seeing someone else and alleging abuse. I told Robert it was important not to get inside her head. It is a good thing we don't really understand what drives true NPDs. If we were to understand them, we would have to be one ourselves. I remind him to think about what he did not receive from his relationship with RR.

This would lead him away from being a victim and towards being back in control.

I could go on and on and on about very severe cases. One of the worst things is that NPDs can destroy someone's values so readily. They tap into a codependent's vulnerable states and kindnesses and extract every ounce of reasonability and value. Sometimes, an NPD will access therapy to justify their actions or reinforce their fantasy. If the therapist is well-trained and experienced and, therefore, knows what they're doing, they would never accept an NPD as a patient through to the end of formulation (unless they just want to collect payment). However, if a codependent accesses a similar therapist, they could help them out of the codependency. But the work is tough and rips them inside-out in the process. Much holding and genuine care is needed by the therapist to manage this to completion.

Of course, most victims will just go through the rest of their lives believing that they are awful and that they are responsible for everything bad that happens to them. Not everyone has access to help—or knows how to.

I hope that this case, this person, this situation, ends soon for Robert and that the law will take its course and he will get his monies and ill-gotten gifts returned. Getting his soul unhooked will take longer. There are promising signs that other victims of RR's games may be coming forward to provide evidence. RR's financial transactions may also shed light on the true extent of the deception.

And what about you, if you are reading this as someone caught in your own toxic relationship? What should you take from this? It takes work to leave an NPD but more than that, it takes huge amounts of work and investment to change ourselves so that we remain kind, thoughtful, loving and wonderful—as we are as human beings, as Robert is—while at the same time putting in boundaries and understanding that to say "no" is not necessarily being mean.

Finally, what alarmed me the most was seeing the contract between Robert and RR. Yes, there was a US$150,000 sports car in the Cayman Islands, a US$400,000 diamond engagement ring, this, that and the other, but the most shocking thing was the condition that Robert moves his entire will, after 18 months of marriage, over to her. That's what an NPD does. They are leeches and won't stop until they have absolutely everything.

That is a huge fortune but that's not the worst of it. How safe would Robert's life be after the 18 months if they had gone ahead? The only way, of course, the NPD would get the will proceeds is if he died! No, this is not fiction. And Robert was so hooked, he signed and agreed to this!

It was an absolutely chilling detail. My gut rolled over. I have been working with Robert for several years. He's a very nice and genuine guy. He says it the way it is, and his kindness and his care and his heart are all in the right place. Unfortunately, he placed his heart with an abuser. Not a scammer or a con artist but an NPD, which is very different. An NPD feeds off people, like a parasite, until they have everything.

And that's why we named this case 'Black Widow' because, like the spider, she will copulate with her partner and then eat him. And that is exactly what she attempted to do.

The colour of hope
One ordinary day, in Robert's log cabin in the mountains, he was feeling tired but also had a strange, deep feeling of impending change.

Earlier, he had had an important session with me and the outcome was yes, let's be on the attack to nail RR but, at the same time, let's keep you safe. Block her numbers, email and any way she can reach you.

So, it came as a shock to Robert's lawyers and I to discover that he had secretly unblocked RR and had recently received messages and calls from her (which, fortunately, he did not respond to). The lead lawyer told Robert to "block now!" I told Robert we needed to protect him and asked him what the point was of 'nailing' her if he was not safe in the process.

Robert was approaching this defence, fight and recovery from evil with precise chess moves but his pattern was to then smash the board, to come out of denial and straight into rage. It gave us all an opportunity to sit back and rethink our approach and reflect on our lack of real understanding about how this NPD could be so unfeeling, cold and venomous. The incomprehensibly powerful nature of this Black Widow had been realised over and over again. New strategies and huge amounts of time were being absorbed in the fight. Everyone was on full alert.

Then, surprisingly, that very evening, when worry for Robert was at a peak, the lawyers and I received pictures. They were of the biggest rainbow crossing the sky in front of Robert's wooden bench where he was having dinner. He sent several of these, explaining that the rainbow was getting brighter and brighter. The pictures kept coming.

A miracle happened that evening. Hope seeped back in. Robert was seeing and feeling the world in a brighter and more vibrant way than ever before in his lifetime. His food tasted just a little better, his favourite rosé wine tasted just that bit crisper. Robert was waking up from his deepest, darkest place.

It was on that evening, at that moment, that Robert finally felt he would make it; he was back in control; he had choices. In fact, he wouldn't just make it but he was on the road to greater things.

This is my purest reward. A soul saved and a soul brighter and more alive. We cannot plan healing, recovery and mending. It comes like an infant comes, "When it is good and ready." Robert was good and ready.

As I sit here writing this, a smile of relief and pride is spreading across my face. Although many souls are lost to the evil of NPD, we have to hold on to the ones we save, the ones we save from themselves. We are on a journey towards the future. I can now rest a little and navigate a path with Robert towards further healing, helping him to put in safeguards to keep him safe from future deadly decisions. Robert still has a lot of repairing to do, a lot of work we need to complete but things are becoming more manageable.

The battle with the legal contracts will continue. We hope that the criminal system may also become involved as the legal case develops. Should this be seen as a crime? Yes, without a doubt. Hopefully this account will one day help with that process.

VV: prey—or predator?

Yet, there could be more twists and turns in this case due to the shadowy role of VV. I initially thought that VV was another victim caught in the Black Widow's trap, deceived by her fake stories of abuse and victimisation. His resources to be used as an accessory to her crimes.

But when this self-professed American Royalty member

and owner of a sports team sent a multi-page letter painting a derogatory picture of Robert, a person whom he has never met, I began to have second thoughts. In this letter, VV displayed his power, implying he was part of a resourceful elite, which included the likes of President Obama and well-known celebrities. Indeed, VV does operate in these circles but why would he use that to give his attack of Robert weight and protect RR?

Is he really a puppet in this case or is he the puppeteer, pulling RR's strings in order to increase his wealth at Robert's expense? And if so, what danger is RR in? After all, a narcissist does not share power with anybody.

RR has also somehow hired one of the top arbitration lawyers in the US and is racking up millions of dollars in fees. The D.C. lawyers have stated they are doing this without deposit or payment of fees as of yet. So, how did RR persuade this legal firm to do this? Is VV involved? Is she luring VV into another web of deceit and lies, or is VV another scheming narcissist, open-eyed and complicit in the deceit? Should VV be warned of RR's capabilities? Or vice versa?

What of her poor children in all of this? Sadly, I am powerless to help. It is time for clinical supervision. Not being able to be a voice for those two innocent children breaks me.

This account has catalogued the systematic attempt of an NPD (and now maybe two NPDs) to destroy somebody. It has been told from my perspective as an experienced therapist supporting a codependent client. But what's going on inside the mind of the NPD herself? How does somebody become so twisted? What internal voices do they hear? What cold messages drive them on?

Inside a narcissist's mind: a true case of dangerous NPD development

A very powerful move I make with people coming out of a toxic relationship is exploring the fact that the narcissist does not think like them. When a kind person makes a move to leave or stand up for themselves, they often start to feel guilty or horrid because they feel they are not caring enough for the narcissist.

In writing this chapter, my plan is to help you understand that the narcissist's blood runs very different to yours. Don't forget that an NPD is developed due to either an over-indulgent childhood, where they believe the world and its souls are there to serve them, or (as in this case) by the most horrific childhood during which they needed to create a fantasy world to survive. Again, the souls of this world are only there to serve them by keeping that image and fantasy intact.

Although we will all feel terrible for RR's start in this world, she could have used her experience for the common good. For whatever reason (we can't know precisely why), she followed her NPD instincts and chose an indulgent and abusive pathway. Remember, with zero remorse or empathy, there is no learning. No recovery.

RR grew up in The Bronx. Her mother left her when she was little so her dad brought her up. Being half Indian was not a helpful start for poor RR. Being adorned with braces, pigtails and glasses was not helpful either. Bullying and being different were unbelievably painful and she was lonely. Desperately lonely. So painful in fact that she learned to hide and even detach from her feelings. No one would know that the piercing racist remarks would hurt like a thousand knives. Being rejected and excluded from a playground game or sports line-up tugged at her stomach as unbearable grief. Fear of school, fear of walking home. Nowhere was safe. Nothing was safe. No one was safe. Becoming an adult felt unreal. No mum or friend to give guidance. Hair sprouting. A fuzzy moustache developing on her upper lip. More targets for fun-making and ridicule. She wet the bed until her mid-teenage years.

Dad was a tough and strict parent but he seemed nice and different when he touched her; something that felt very wrong and scary to her. Part of RR died when this started. She'd freeze. Feel sickened and barely able to breathe. She'd never show it though. RR's only escape was to dream of a different world. A world far from the dark and desperate walls of her childhood.

TV was her parent, her educator, her lifeline. She'd dress up in secret and try to imitate the 'beautiful people.' She often caught the subway across to Manhattan where she would visit the Upper East Side and watch how the wealthy people behaved: the way they would greet and sit and talk. The wealthy Ivy League students were always smiling. RR would often go home and practice smiling in the mirror, greeting fictitious friends as she had observed. Prancing up and down in her bedroom looking at herself in the long mirror. Pulling her shoulders back and forcing her chin up. She was always surprised at how different she would look by posing and making her face different. There was nothing she could do about her nose though; she hated this inherited lump on her face. She used sticky tape at times to try to change it but hiding it with a scarf would sometimes do the trick.

Eating was RR's comfort too. Along with puppy fat came the result of hot dogs, burgers and other local delicacies that did not necessarily agree with her budding ambition of being a well-heeled, popular lady, film star or model. Someone that could command good service and the recognition of being above par at bars and restaurants. This became RR's obsession. She'd practice and practice in her room. If she were going to escape this place she needed to work on a way out.

RR did moderately well at school but trying to survive took the edge off what she may have achieved. She was bright enough but due to the schooling in the area she was brought up in, she never learnt the classics or grammar and she had the Bronx accent. At 16, she got a Saturday job in the local mall and made a few acquaintances. She became fascinated to learn that some of the girls would go to parties and bars in New York City. Looking a little older, she started to get the train to New York herself, craving the big city and the fast pace there. Going through a growth spurt and getting out more, RR slimmed down. With a little help from her friend's makeup collection, she noticed that she was attracting some attention from boys.

She met a boy on one of her nights out in NYC and they started dating. She enjoyed sex with him and realised that her body was quite a powerful tool.

'I want to bring my dreams of wealth to life,' she thinks. 'If sex has this effect over one powerless boy, surely I can use it to hook up with the rich and powerful.'

Stepping outside RR's world for a moment, we can most easily get an insight into a narcissist's mind by inserting quotations to symbolise thought processes. We can't, of course, know exactly what words were silently spoken by RR but I have had enough experience of NPDs (including RR herself) through my codependent patients (plus evidence from letters, emails, recorded messages, etc) to make educated assumptions. The point here is to show how RR is already making her plans to discard her first victim as she builds her perfect life—an island far away from her abusive upbringing. The further the better.

RR swiftly discarded the boy and moved on to the next and the next and the next. She started to meet new friends on the New York party scene. She started to smoke and take poppers, barbiturates and cocaine. All helped with her confidence and weight. It was not long until RR started to get drinks and meals from leering men at dance clubs. One night, a new 'friend' introduced her to a scout for a pole dancing club and she soon had a regular gig at the club where she cavorted with some of New York's most influential and elite.

RR left school and used the pole dancing money to move into a shared apartment in NYC. But she was soon to realise that there was a ceiling to this work. Lap dancing was lucrative and powerful but she knew there was more, better. This way she was not integrated or part of the elite; she was the 'dirty secret.' She soon found a way to polish up her act and found work at the more prestigious bars. But what of her story? Elite people went to Ivy League colleges and looked and spoke well. She needed to learn, change it up.

RR had a nose reconstruction and applied for college, getting a place on a catering course. She learnt the best way to serve and cook, to present tables, to greet and talk with people. The makeup counters in New York helped her with a more subtle and polished look. After a few years of stashing her lap dance money and completing college, she took off to Europe, to Florence, Italy, to start a new life, 'Louis Vuitton,' plastic, made-in-China bag in tow. One of the girls had married and moved there with her husband.

RR's savings went quite far because the currency was cheaper but her focus was on targeting a man of status who would give her the image and lifestyle she longed for. After all, RR now polished up well and resembled a respectable and acceptable well-heeled lady. She went out with her friend and developed a very charming and almost mystical image. In fact, she found that she could completely reinvent herself. She was learning Italian and her story was that she took a break from studying and wanted some space from her family. She was always careful to protect their identity and her own.

So, with her Italian coming along nicely, she dated here and there until one night she struck gold. A good looking man with a good job took her to dinner. She had learned not to give too much on the first date, as ladies did not do that. Instead, she played with him—and he fell for her. She left him and found that the more she left him the more he wanted her. 'This is quite a fun game,' RR thought. 'Let's see what I can get out of him.' The 'relationship' was on and off for a year but it was not enough. He was not enough. She saw bigger and better.

Besides, Florence was too small. With her catering and service training, a new chic style from Italy (as well as a command of the language) and one real statement handbag, she returned to America and headed to Chicago, fresh off the plane with a new story: of university in Italy not finished, of leaving a bad relationship there (but couldn't talk about it as he was a VIP).

She frequented the bars and private clubs and studied the men there. One evening she heard a chap speaking in Italian. She chirped in and the rest is history.

She married the Italian stockbroker who was mesmerised by her looks, who took pity on her over her hint of a story. They soon had a child. Her only mistake was that she didn't realise even he could not keep up with her exorbitant lifestyle demands. Clothes, shoes, nanny, meals, trips, they all took a toll not to mention their hefty mortgage. In an attempt to keep up, he succumbed to fraudulent trading and was caught and fired, ruining her image. 'How dare he do this to me?' RR raged. Even though he soon become employed again, his job was even less lucrative. 'Time to go up a level,' RR thought.

RR just couldn't be satiated. Equipped with an Italian husband, a house in Lincoln Park and a fake Northeast accent that only an Ivy League alumni could ever try to match, RR was still figuring out how to get more.

RR's husband was depleted and begged her to give him a chance. He apologised and, like a good codependent, tried to make everything right again. 'Stick around if you have to then,' she thought. 'You might be useful.' A spider knows when to wait and when to strike!

She found an elite dating agency in Chicago and made an appointment with Clare, the owner. She explained that she was divorced and with a child. She gave Clare her Lincoln Park address and explained that she was educated and spoke Italian. As RR presented herself so well, Clare gave her membership. Clare received up to US$100,000 from her gentlemen members and US$5,000 a pop for each introduction. RR could hardly contain her glee when Clare explained that there was no end to the men she could introduce her to. Within a few months, RR had met and was dating 12 men with Clare's blessing. Clare groomed RR in how to operate. Get them hooked and offer an exclusive. Charge them US$20,000 to US$50,000 per month to keep up with their wealthy lifestyles.

And yes, they mostly agreed.

She had told her codependent husband that his illegal trading had got them into this mess and if he wanted her and their child to stay in Chicago, he needed to help her put things right. In fear of losing RR and his child, he agreed to support her agency career. He even helped keep portfolios on each man, and to take sexy but safe pictures of RR, so that she could see them rarely but keep them keen.

She made nearly US$1.7 million in her first two years. Not to mention bags, jewellery and other gifts, all easily saleable, for another US$500,000 or so. It was an elaborate plan spearheaded by RR and actively supported by her husband who realised there was money to be made.

Of course, as with all scams there was bound to be a hiccup. RR and her husband were doing so well for themselves that they had become careless, going on family holidays together. This made her exclusive dating agreements complicated. Some of the men were getting suspicious. She needed a reasonable way to break off some of these relationships. 'I've always liked the idea of two children,' she thought, 'If I get pregnant now, I can get rid of some of the wasters.'

There was one man she wanted to keep interested. Although he was on the older side, he had offered RR the world. What's more, he was clearly a bit green to the dating scene, having recently come out of a long-term marriage. He had given her an in-door to private clubs and a generous offer of a prenuptial, an agreement worth one million up front.

When she did fall pregnant, RR spun a story about the

second child being conceived by IVF and all because she remembered being such a lonely child and didn't want this for her child. She explained that medically it would be better to have two children from the same father in case there was ever an issue. Well, he was sucked in and forgave her and she now almost had the perfect set up.

She still needed a way to escape her marriage though and divorce was an expense she would rather avoid. So, as she filed for divorce and briefed her lawyers to strip her husband of everything, she got some of the men she was dating to pay her legal bills. 'I've been so abused by him,' she would cry, becoming quite the expert at turning on the water-works. 'You need to support and protect me.' Her vulnerable beauty won them over every time.

She did divorce her husband, and he moved into a separate apartment, but she was not quite done with him yet. There were benefits of living a fake life as man and wife, complete with luxury marital home. So she spent a lot of time with her ex even as she 'moved in' with Robert.

But an NPD is never satisfied and is always alert, ready to catch the next big fish.

Whilst in Portofino with Robert on their yacht, RR ran into an American match-maker while visiting a hotel. An elite and very exclusive match-maker, she had read Robert and RR's situation perfectly. They became the best of friends after three hours of talking. The plan was agreed. RR was to meet a billionaire (VV) but it needed to be the very next week. That could be done. RR explained to Robert that she needed to go to a friend's birthday party in San Francisco and would take the children to Chicago with the two nannies she travelled with. From there, she was to pop over to San Francisco for a few days. Unsuspecting Robert agreed, of course, even giving her the private jet to Chicago and then a First Class AA ticket to San Francisco. Who wouldn't believe this tale?

Then Robert threw a spanner in the works when his son had an accident en route to Portofino. Without an ounce of empathy for Robert and his son, RR slipped into a narcissistic rage. "You had better be careful," she screamed. "There are bigger fish in the sea than you." Not realising that these words had finally roused Robert's suspicions, she went ahead to reel VV in. Even as she entered the security code to access VV's home, she was being secretly tracked.

She was genuinely shocked when a stranger handed her a note from Robert whilst she was sitting opposite VV in a classy restaurant. She knew it was from Robert as he had used her pet name. He was breaking up with her, which was irritating. It was too soon to move on from Robert as she hadn't secured his will. That meant she would have to win him back all over again by sending him seductive images, messages of how sorry she was and promises that she would make it up to him.

She admitted the fling but promised it was all over. Little did Robert know that the real issue was that VV was not as generous as he had been. Although he had proposed marriage, he was not putting enough up front (RR was realising why his nickname was 'Alligator Arms'—always the last to lean forward for the bill at the restaurant!). Still, time was on her side.

Robert was over the moon. RR had her assurance of US$5.5 million within a month of engagement in Paris. There was then to be a nine-month cohabitation to end in a summer wedding. And 18 months after marriage, Robert's will—his whole world—would be hers. But Robert was not nearly as wealthy as VV. Nor did he operate in the same elite political and billionaire circles. VV was now offering her the world and a full life with him in San Francisco—for her and her two children—and his world was a lot bigger than Robert's!

RR did everything she could to not be with Robert. He was in the Cayman Islands and for tax reasons, had limited days he could be in the US. He gave RR the option to move to the Caymans with him but she used the children and umpteen other reasons to refuse. When he was in the US, she would spend most of her time with her husband stating she had business to attend to. She spent a lot of the rest of the time talking with VV. He was offered her too much status to turn down. The people in the Upper East Side were nothing in comparison to this. She had no more use for her husband or Robert but she would stay and collect the cohab money. 'That will give me around seven million of my own,' she calculated. 'With my own stash, I won't need as much security from VV. Besides, the money is rightfully mine.'

That is how she thinks. She has no issues around Robert's feelings or the welfare of her children, whom she sees only occasionally. And once she is in San Francisco, she will be eyeing the people at the very top, finding ways to topple VV, as she climbs the ladder. After all, the bigger they are, the harder they fall. Unless she has unwittingly wandered into a trap of her own. VV has already displayed a ruthless, malicious and bullying streak as he threatens Robert with the might of his connections.

RR's story could be coming to its conclusion. She may believe her ideal world is within her grasp. It would be a tragic irony if she were to end up stripped of her power and at the mercy of a ruthless abuser.

This is a slight insight into an NPD's thinking. It is cold and calculated. Other humans exist purely for their use. The NPD needs ever-increasing wealth, like a drug addict always needs a bigger fix of drugs, to be satisfied. Think of this very real case the next time you feel sorry for—or sad about—your NPD. They are excellent actors. Their whole mission is to feed their lifestyle and self-image. They are convincing because they believe their own story.

Not all narcissists climb the ladder as efficiently as RR. This is a particularly glamorous and wealthy case but, whatever context you are in, the narcissist will be equally cold, deceitful and toxic.

Just think, if RR hadn't chanced upon that Italian in Chicago, who knows where she would have been hatching her next plot, spinning her deadly webs.

PART II

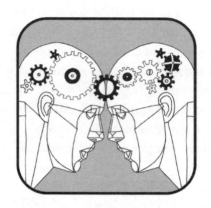

DIFFERENT PERSPECTIVES: NARCISSISM AND CODEPENDENCY OUTSIDE OF THERAPY

"If you judge people, you have no time to love them."
-Mother Teresa-

CHAPTER 7

FOUR UNIQUE LENSES

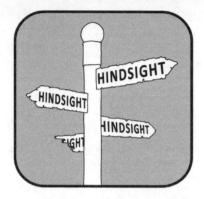

*"Hindsight Hell is what you're entering
when you're starting to question your life decisions."*
-Michael Padraig Acton-

As explained in the introduction, I wanted to dedicate part of this book to understanding how professionals in different fields experience the narcissism-codependent dynamic. From the courtroom and the accountant's office to the paediatrician's clinic and the life coach's room, the same pattern rears its head but in very different contexts.

If you are a codependent, you may pick up valuable hints from this chapter as to what lies ahead of you during a court battle, divorce mediation, child's health issue or life coaching work.

I will duly stand aside for the duration of this chapter and invite four esteemed contributors to step forward to the podium and reveal how codependency and narcissism looks from their viewpoint.

NO ACCOUNTING FOR NARCISSISTS
By Loretta Fabricant, CPA, CFF ABV Fabricant and co.

As a Forensic accountant, I have been involved in more than 5,000 divorces in my 40 years of practice. I have had the opportunity to encounter NPDs at their worst (if you can imagine that)!

The discovery phase: During the discovery phase of my work, I need my clients to gather documents relative to their income, expenses, assets and liabilities. Getting information out of an NPD client is like pulling teeth! They are always quick to say that their spouse knows all this information and to ask if they really need to produce all of these records. I have noticed, fairly consistently, the codependent spouse doing the financial discovery work for the NPD.

The NPD client believes that rules are for other people, not them, and cannot understand why I don't just take their word for the value of their assets or income. They also believe that their own spending is minimal and their spouse is the big spender.

I have sometimes had to show my client the hard proof that they are in fact the bigger spender, which is when they share all of their valid reasons for spending that much.

The NPD personality will be glad to tell you that they were the only one who ever brought anything to the marriage. They don't think that their partner of however many years deserves anything and the thought that if their ex-wives live well, so will their children, never occurs to them. There is no empathy and no sympathy.

However, they are more than happy to tell me how terrible their spouse is and how outraged they are that they are putting them through this.

Where my client is the codependent spouse of someone with NPD, I have seen them brainwashed to the point that they believe the narcissist more than their own professionals. I then have to fight with my own client to get them to see reality!

In all aspects of their divorce, the narcissist is now the star of a movie about them. They like the attention and feel they are controlling the situation. They are very charming until you tell them something they do not want to hear, like how the law works or that they have to pay alimony or give the other side some documents. Then the demon comes out! As with the discovery documents, the NPD believes all they have to do is tell you something and that should be enough—no proof necessary—they have spoken!

The settlement phase: When it comes to the settlement portion of the divorce, one very important factor that impacts everything is. . . who wanted out? If the person with NPD asked for the divorce, then there is steady movement forward.

However, if the codependent spouse had finally had enough and chose to divorce, there is all hell to pay. Narcissists are not done with you until they say they are! I have been involved with cases that, even after the divorce, the person with NPD files motion after motion in order to torment their ex-spouse. In Tennessee, the legislation actually passed a rule where judges must look at the entire file in divorce cases to see if the person with NPD is harassing the ex-spouse!

The mediation phase: In most cases, mediation is the last stage of the litigation; only about 10% of divorces actually have to be tried.

Mediation is the place where the narcissist shines and his or her true colours come out in all their glory. In mediation, he or she can be the star and the manipulator in charge. There, the psychology specialists, lawyers and financial experts all have to figure out a way to placate the person with NPD into doing the right thing. This is really hard work. If one thing is suggested that the narcissist didn't come up with, they gets up and are ready to leave.

During the eight to 12 hours of mediation, everyone walks on eggshells trying to reach a reasonable settlement while not upsetting the person with NPD.

There are about four hours at least of back and forth over what they can and can't agree to. Another four hours is spent listening to why the narcissist is the victim and the soon to be former spouse should get nothing!

At the end of the day, most NPD cases do not settle and the professionals walk away frustrated, exhausted, and feeling like they have just competed in the Olympics and finished in fourth place! In order to end the madness, the codependent often winds up taking less than they deserve just to buy peace which is, as the Mastercard commercial reads, priceless.

COURTING DISASTER
By Sarah Zabel, Former Circuit Court Judge, Maze Resolutions PA

Divorce, finance and power struggles in court: I don't want to be gender specific but I will say that in many of the divorce cases I presided over, the husband had total control over all of the finances and total control over the wife.

I think it's important, in relation to what this book is about, to say that in many of these cases, women had given up their careers. For example, they might have got their law degree but never practised law. Instead, they stayed at home, raised the children and put their faith in marriage vows. Then, all of a sudden, the marriage imploded. It may have been because of an extra-marital affair or the marriage just didn't work out.

These women would often come into court with nothing and you could observe the eye contact and body language. I'm not a psychologist or therapist but you didn't have to be a professional to see the difference between one side and the other. One would be more dominant because they had control of the purse strings.

Whether or not that made that person a narcissist, or the other person a codependent, I would have to defer that to the professionals. But just as an observation from me, being on the bench, you could see the power struggle.

Where one side is unable to access financial accounts how are they supposed to pay for an attorney or cover their living expenses? To pay for a mortgage or an apartment?

They have given themselves for years to one person, turned everything over to that one person, raised their children and, all of a sudden, the floor collapses from under them and they're lost.

In many cases, where one side could not access accounts, lawyers would have to run into court getting money and support. The other side knew they had the leverage and all they had to do was wait it out. They would postpone things and make things difficult, so that the person would just cave in and agree to take less than maybe they should have based on all the years of marriage.

I guess a lot of people think, in this day and age, that this doesn't happen because a lot of women are now in the workforce. But in the cocoon of the family court system it happens a lot and you can see the dejection with those who are not in a position of control.

There have been accounts where women hold the purse strings but not in the majority of cases. . . although I think the trend is changing.

The courtroom as a stage for the narcissist: I once had a very interesting paternity case. The man had a relationship with two women and all three lived together.

They all worked and were well educated but, in the relationship, the man was dominant over the two women. Both women had babies at the same time but one of them felt she needed to break out otherwise she was going to lose herself.

There was a paternity case filed and the man, who eventually married the woman who stayed with him, came to court. Without disrespecting him, you could see the difference in eye contact between the pair; she would look down while his whole aura was concerned with trying to control the courtroom. She was more passive and while he was not aggressive in a physical way, his whole demeanour was certainly very assertive.

He was monopolising the space in the room but she also had a very good lawyer so things didn't always go his way.

Sometimes you can be your own worst enemy, as they say. That case certainly stands out to me.

The invisible scars of domestic abuse: Not all victims of domestic violence live on the poverty line. Many are educated, professional women but you can't see the scars because they're invisible. With physical abuse, you can see the scars from the outside but you can't see the terrible emotional abuse somebody's going through within the confines of their own home and that's true for children too.

It becomes a vicious cycle because, in a lot of cases, children who are abused grow up to become abusers themselves.

Without proper intervention, whether that is individual therapy, family therapy or other resources to break that cycle, it just continues.

The abuser takes the victim and brings them down to a level where they are paralysed and cannot escape. It becomes a sick kind of love because the victim thinks they still love this abuser and can't live beyond them. Until they 100% cut that cord, they are still tied to the person and can't see what's right in front of them: that they've been knocked down and the abuser has brought them down to such a degree that they can't function.

I think the abusers themselves are dysfunctional. For some of them, the abusive control is a twisted way of saying they love that person. Afterwards they apologise, but it's a sickness.

On the other hand, I've handled a lot of domestic violence cases, when I was in court and even now as a mediator, where somebody uses the court system to file a frivolous domestic violence case in order to get a one up on their custody case.

This is just horrible because it takes time away from people who actually need the system.

The use and misuse of labels in court: I find that labels can be overused and some people like to come into court and use those labels as a reason to control the situation. For example, there may be an allegation that one parent is narcissistic or bipolar.

But just because you are diagnosed bipolar, and I defer to the professionals of course, it doesn't mean that you can't function and be a good parent. The opposite is also true: if you don't have a diagnosed condition it doesn't mean that you are a good parent.

In a divorce case, a couple might have been married for years and everything was perfect. Then, all of a sudden, things implode and now one person is labelling the other person narcissistic or bipolar in order to be in control or to have a one up in their court case. They are using the court system but it's the judges and lawyers who should be taking the lead. Sometimes, the clients are driving the bus which, in one respect, is correct but lawyers also have to control their clients. They have an ethical duty to present the case and not bring something to the court that's frivolous. There's a fine line.

If a client is going to their lawyer saying the other person is narcissistic, bipolar or incompetent to take care of the children, or to hold on to the financial resources, the lawyers then need to come into court, file the necessary motions and really make things messier than they should be. Lawyers should take their clients with a grain of salt while representing them to the best of their ability.

Lawyers might come into court and ask for a psychological evaluation but there's a certain threshold that they have to cross. They have to bring it in good faith, they have to have a hearing and then the court has to evaluate the circumstances and make a decision about whether to order an evaluation or not.

Sometimes they look at the background too. The individual may have already gone through therapy and received a diagnosis, or they might be on some type of psychotropic medication that would lead to an evaluation being granted. Sometimes there are other factors taken into consideration like drug abuse. Has that person been bankrupted?

Has that person had some type of breakdown? Is the individual able to make conscious decisions?

Just because one side says that there needs to be a psychological evaluation, that's not the threshold. You have to have factual information.

Courts should be very conscious of what kind of psychological evaluation is granted. Sometimes, one side is going on a fishing expedition to try and cherry pick things they can use against the other side, so it might be decided to order a limited evaluation to determine, for example, whether alienation is occurring. That can be interesting because narcissistic tendencies and other things within the psychology of the alienator can come up. Again, I'm not a psychologist but I've seen a lot of these evaluations and sometimes recognise that one parent is trying to keep the child away from the other and destroy that relationship.

They don't want the other parent to co-parent because they want to keep the child to themselves. It's not 'we', it's 'I' and it's unfortunate but it happens more often than not.

The goal is often 'win at all costs' and unfortunately, the only ones who end up losing are the children, whether or not their parents are narcissists, bipolar or whatever. This is the family court system.

Narcissism and the rise in elder abuse: In some cases, adult children, who may be narcissists or have other psychological issues, use financial methods, for example power of attorney, as a control over their elderly parents.

This dynamic is the polar opposite to the one where you have a child or children going through the court system where one parent might be a narcissist and the other a codependent.

I once had a case involving a couple in their seventies. The husband wanted a divorce but really what was behind it was the older children and it had to do with money. One sibling was with the mother and the other with the father and they were controlling the situation to the point where the father petitioned for the dissolution of a more than 40 year marriage.

These people were living on fixed incomes and were relying on their children who they trusted. It's just like the domestic violence cases where one person puts their trust in the other and that person abuses that trust.

These elderly people had raised and taken care of their children and now their children were taking advantage of their parents instead of taking care of them during their golden age where life is not long. That's very sad and very tragic.

A warning on family courts, mental health and lost childhood: Family court is the last place families should be because litigation changes people! The sooner you resolve cases and the more you can keep people out of the family court system the better because the more they continue the more they unravel.

I could see people unravelling because they couldn't take the anxiety and the stress of the unknown, especially where custody and time sharing is concerned.

Whether their parents are narcissists or not, once children are brought into the court system, it becomes toxic. There is alienation, where visitations are frustrated and there's the 'dangling the carrot over the head' situation in which one side holds back child support because the other side isn't letting them visit the child. The power struggle is between the two parents but the child or the children are right in the middle.

I want to mention post-traumatic stress disorder. Being in the family court system is very traumatic and for children, the scars do not heal. If they are evaluated, in many cases they are diagnosed with PTSD.

The longer they are put through the court system and experience the custody battle between the parents, the more it affects their relationships as they grow up. It can affect the relationships in their employment and their relationships with a significant other because they don't know what a healthy relationship is. They only know that toxic relationship between their parents.

I think the age where children are most affected is between seven and 13. Very young children and babies haven't developed to the stage where it's going to impact them while older children are more independent. They have already gone through puberty and understand who they are. It's those in between ages between seven and 13, especially where children are going through puberty, that are so hard.

These children are still forming their own identities and now there are these other factors that are destroying their ability to function in school or to have a healthy relationship with friends. Their parents are taking up all the space in their lives, their childhood goes by very quickly and now they're adults but can't have healthy relationships with other adults because of what their parents put them through.

I once had a post-judgment case where one parent was a doctor and the other a successful businessman. Money was a non-issue but one parent wanted their child to go to public school and the other parent wanted their child to go to private school and they wanted me to make that decision.

A judge shouldn't have to make a decision over what school a child should go to but when you have that power struggle, sometimes the dysfunction is so extreme that neither parent can agree in a healthy way for what is in the best interest of their child. It's crazy, I know and that's just the tip of the iceberg!

I tell parents who are going through a divorce; you may be divorcing as a couple but you will never divorce as parents. The healthiest co-parenting relationship is where you take that parenting plan, you shove it in a drawer and you never use it.

PERSONAL AGENCY
By Jim Davis, Ontological, Ecological and Mindfulness Coach

Once I got introduced to transformation work and self-development, I was hooked. I think it's a gift to be able to give someone the space to explore possibilities and create new horizons.

The challenge of working with narcissists and codependents: As a life coach, I work with people who really step into their agency and effectiveness.

With a narcissist, it's about how do you assert yourself, be effective and also allow the space for others to show up as themselves? To not be the only one to the party? Are they willing to really take a hard look at themselves, make changes and be honest and authentic with themselves?

For codependents, I would want them to really hone in on what is and isn't working, and what they are looking to get out of our work together. Clearly, they're coming to me for new answers and new possibilities.

But when someone is codependent, their life has become hinged on someone else's approval or life so they don't have their full agency, their full authorship to bring forth their own life.

I think that the biggest pain a human can feel is an assault on their dignity. That's really what a narcissist does. People want to have their dignity and they want to feel like they are someone who co-creates. When that doesn't happen, that's when the pain happens.

Is a codependent willing to commit to stepping into their full power? Because if they're on the fence then it really becomes a very difficult challenge and perhaps therapy or something like that might be a better venture for them. It just depends on where they are in their situation.

Hitting rocks: from failure to acceptance: We have all the tools necessary to live life so it's a matter of what is in our toolbox that's effective for us when we hit rocks?

How can we make that turn and stop hitting the rock? What I find is that people continue to hit the rock because there's no space for a new possibility. Coaching allows someone to create that new possibility.

First of all, you have to believe in your abilities to navigate life. You have to have an effective belief system because if you think that you deserve the rock then that's what you'll have.

One thing in my particular coaching is that there are no failures, only feedback. When you can really embrace that distinction, it allows you to navigate through life without this heaviness. It allows you to say, 'This is the experience of life', versus 'This is me'. Facts versus interpretations. This is what happened and this is what I made up about it.

Personal agency is also about the boundaries and agreements you have with yourself and those that you communicate with other people. It's about having that sovereignty when approaching any relationship or co-creation and having it actually be a co-creation versus losing yourself. Utilising boundaries and agreements sets the tone and provides support, much like ground rules.

My top advice: My top advice, for both narcissists and codependents, is to learn acceptance. Learn to accept who you are, even those parts that you judge are weak or not congruent. If you can become accepting of your 'shortcomings' and of situations that arise, you can take responsibility for them. And not responsibility as a way to blame yourself but as a guide to how to respond (respond, responsibility, same words) and as a gateway to your own personal freedom, agency, peace and joy.

MOTHER KNOWS BEST
By Barry Scott Lowy, MD Paediatrician

I have had the pleasure of working with a mother and son who together offered me the experience to work with the NPD and codependent relationship.

When I met the mother, she made a separate appointment to discuss her concerns about her 18-year-old son. Her statements were a matter of fact and of a dire nature. Her speech was pressured and the anguish in her face was real. I sat quietly as she spoke continuously unless I created a pause to explore further. When I did try to pause the conversation, I was met with a great deal of resistance. It was very important that she was heard and believed and it was implausible that she had this wrong. She needed me to speak with her son right away and would take whatever actions necessary.

As her family paediatrician, I took her concerns seriously and we scheduled an appointment for her son so he could come and see me independent of her. The following day, the son showed up with mum. At first, the son was sitting alone in the room with mum in the waiting room. To me, this was the best scenario to create a safe space for him to talk about why he was here.

Well, our private conversation lasted less than two-and-a-half minutes before the mother barged in to the room proclaiming that she had been standing outside the door and that her son was lying and making up stories to purposely make her look wrong.

His demeanour changed instantly as his shoulders slumped, his eyes went to looking at the floor and he stopped talking.

Once again, the mother went on with a well-scripted and rehearsed monologue. The son sat there powerless and seemed to start crying. He regained his voice but continued to look downward. Their topic was about him applying to college and which one he should go to. Typically, a family discussion about this topic occurs with proper guidance from the parent or parents who would be making a concerted effort to create an outcome of their child's choice. This was not the case with this parent and son. Despite several appointments, the outcome had similar results with the son made to feel inferior, that his opinion was wrong and that he was not thinking right. Mother made it very clear that her opinion was correct and that she needed me to support her in having him see her point of view.

RECOMMENDED READING

Addiction, Narcissism, Divorce-Haley Thompson

Narcissism and Manipulation-Dr Isabel M. Brown

Splitting: Protecting Yourself While Divorcing Someone with Narcissistic Personality Disorder-Bill Eddy and Randi Kreger

How to Divorce a Narcissist or a Psychopath-Sam Vaknin and Lidija Rangelovska

Divorcing A Narcissist-Covert Harper J.

Disarming the Narcissist: How to Stay Married to a Narcissistic Partner and Be (Reasonably) Happy-Nora Simpson, Maureen McLain, et al.

Will I Ever Be Free of You? How to Navigate a High-Conflict Divorce from a Narcissist and Heal Your Family-Dr Karyl McBride ph.D.

A Divorce Companion-The Best of the Great Escape: Divorce Topics from Narcissism to Financial Recovery to Sex and Love-Lisa Thomson

Credit, Cash and Codependency: The Money Connection-Yvonne Kaye and Daniel Sean Kaye

Exposing Financial Abuse: When Money is a Weapon-Shannon Thomas LCSW

How to Annihilate a Narcissist: In the Family Court-Rachel Watson

Divorcing a Narcissist: One Mom's Battle-Tina Swithin

Parental Alienation Syndrome: Child Brainwashing Hacks Used by Narcissists (in 30 Minutes)-J.B. Snow, Gene Blake, et al.

Trapped in the Mirror: Adult Children of Narcissists in Their Struggle for Self-Elan Golomb

Healing the Adult Children of Narcissists: Essays on the Invisible War Zone and Exercises for Recovery-Shahida Arabi

Divorcing and Healing from a Narcissist-Dr Theresa J. Covert and Trei Taylor

Narcissistic Mothers-Dr Theresa J. Covert

My Road Beyond the Codependent Divorce-Lisa A. Romano

Out of the Mirror: A Workbook of Healing for Adult Children of Covert Narcissists-Beth McDonald

Narcissistic Parents: The Complete Guide for Adult Children-Caroline Foster and Trei Taylor

The Codependency Recovery Plan: A 5-Step Guide to Understand, Accept, and Break Free from the Codependent Cycle-Krystal Mazzola M.Ed LMFT

Empath, Narcissists and Codependency Cycle Recovery-Daniel Anderson

Rapha's 12-Step Program for Overcoming Codependency-Pat Springle

The Codependency Workbook: Simple Practices for Developing and Maintaining Your Independence-Krystal Mazzola M.Ed LMFT

Codependency Recovery Guide-Joshua Moore

Take Control of Your Life-Daniel Jave and Frank Gerard

Codependent Cure-Jean Harrison and Beattie Grey

Stop Being Codependent in 10 Easy Steps-Catie Grandmaison

Cure Codependency and Conquer as an Empath-Leanne Walters and Carol Grace Anderson

Breaking Codependency: How to Navigate the Traps That Sabotage Your Life-Lesly Devereaux

Narcissistic Disorders in Children and Adolescents: Diagnosis and Treatment-Phyllis Beren

Raising Resilient Children with a Borderline or Narcissistic Parent-Margalis Fjelstad and Jean McBride

Narcissistic Parents: Why Emotionally Immature Parents Infantilise Their Children-Cecilia Overt

Children and Narcissistic Personality Disorder: A Guide for Parents-Cynthia Bailey-Rug

Co-Parenting with a Toxic Ex-Amy J.L. Baker ph.D, Raul R. Fine LCSW, et al.

Dealing with Emotionally Immature Parents: How to Handle Toxic Parents-Priscilla Posey and Robin Howatt Shrock

Narcissistic Mothers-Elizabeth Ex

The Narcissistic Family: Diagnosis and Treatment-Stephanie Donaldson-Pressman and Robert M. Pressman

Narcissistic Mothers-Michelle Evans, Angela Peel, et al.

Education in a Narcissistic Nation: Build Foundations for Students, Not Pedestals-Karen Brackman and Chad Mason

CHAPTER 8

MANAGING CODEPENDENCY IN THE WORKPLACE

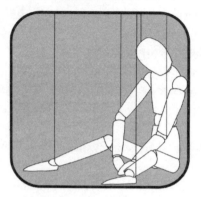

"Work stress kills more than just your personal life."
-Michael Padraig Acton-

As Jackie mentioned in an earlier case study for this book, "I am not like this at work."

This statement opens up some fascinating areas of exploration, which are hardly ever touched upon in mainstream books about narcissism or codependency. Some of the questions you might have include:

- How does codependency affect work relationships and performance?
- What is it like to work under (or above) a narcissist?
- How can I protect my business or partnership from toxic relationships?
- What happens when a narcissist and a codependent

meet in a work context (e.g. what if John were Jackie's boss?)

At the start of this book, I pointed out an important distinction between narcissistic and codependent traits and NPD or codependency. It is worth emphasising this distinction in this chapter because NPD and codependency only work as a double act. An employee, employer, freelancer or patient with narcissistic or codependent traits always has the potential to enter into a toxic relationship but the context is all important.

Recognising and dealing with codependent traits

If you have codependent traits, you may go overboard to fix problems, work beyond your contracted hours, panic when a customer gets angry, accept a low wage or take on projects you don't enjoy.

However, unless your bosses or clients have narcissistic traits and have a major say in your career or business, you are unlikely to see your life fall apart around you!

A good strategy for dealing with this kind of situation is to listen to your internal dialogue and gently challenge any internal rules that are making you responsible for the emotional state of others. These might include:

- If I make a mistake, I'm useless.
- If someone's angry or upset, I'm to blame and it's my responsibility to make them feel better.
- If someone is in trouble, I should always help them.
- My clients need me because no one else can do this work.
- If they don't like my work, they don't like me

Replace these with:

- Everybody makes mistakes. Every business makes mistakes.
- People are responsible for their own emotional reactions.
- I don't always have to help everyone else out.
- My time is valuable and I choose to give it to people who respect that.
- I believe in my performance/product.

The effect of narcissists in the workplace

We have probably all experienced the narcissistic tyrant in a position of power (as a supervisor or manager). Again, this can be unpleasant and even traumatic but we are unlikely to be in a codependent relationship with them.

Narcissists often make their way to the top in organisations but they are also found among the rank and file. This is rarely a stable situation since narcissists believe that their rightful place is calling the shots.

They will almost always be working to undermine their supervisors and managers and to engineer situations where they are seen as a cut above everyone else.

The NPD and codependency dance at work: a case study

Although it is more difficult to create that all-consuming toxic context in the workplace, it can happen. It must be remembered that someone with codependent traits is always looking to be the provider while the narcissist demands total obedience and unwavering attention.

If a codependent employee hooks up with a narcissist in

the workplace, then the dynamic will kick into play until one or the other cuts the cord.

I know only too well the havoc that inadvertently linking up with a narcissist in the workplace can wreak because it happened to me:

At the time, I really didn't know what narcissism or codependency was. I was in clinical training, working in a hospital, and my clinical consultant was not only my line manager, not only my clinical supervisor but also my external supervisor.

This person could make my life great or terrible and as the weekend loomed I really started to live in fear of how she would be at my clinical supervision, which was always on a Friday.

She could make or break me and I often left her thinking that I was 'bad' and 'wrong' and could never hope to be a psychologist or a therapist. It sounds really awful, but sometimes I was in tears on my way home.

This went on for almost two years and I did everything I could to please this person. Sometimes it was accepted but sometimes it wasn't and I wasn't sure what to do. I definitely wasn't streetwise then and I didn't know how to play the game or even what the game was.

Then, halfway through my thesis, the university explained to me that there were some issues with my external clinical supervisor (which was her). Imagine! I get feedback from the university which can affect my references in the future, my job and my training. It could ruin my degree in Psychology and Education.

I was really trapped. She had so much power over my patient

load, over my conduct as an Assistant Clinical Psychologist and over my position as a student at the university that I felt in front of a firing range—and she could pull the trigger at any time. That's why in therapy and psychology we should never take up dangerous dual roles.

I had to do everything to keep her happy and please her. That's the codependent stance and it became my whole modus operandi.

I went in for my clinical supervision one Friday and she was super sweet and being very familiar and just chit-chatting. I thought it was wonderful at first.

But then she got a little bit closer and I became very uneasy and felt quite nauseous, as if something was wrong.

This woman was probably in her mid to late-50s and always dressed smartly. I was in my early 30s. Things had been said throughout our relationship but I never knew which way to take it. But at this point I thought, 'God, you idiot, she fancies you. Maybe there's been another type of relationship with this!'

In one way it got better for me after that because I could see what was going on. But it also got worse because she realised that I had recognised her motives and was then forced into defending her position as my line manager, as the consultant psychologist in the department and as my external supervisor.

I was then put in another very difficult position when the university told me they were not getting what they needed back from my external supervisor, which of course was her.

I thought my world had ended.

My world was very small at the time: I was a single dad most of the time because the mother of my daughter wasn't very well, I was doing several jobs, I was studying all hours and

I was at the hospital three-and-a-half days a week. I felt sick to the depths of my stomach because I had to ask for a new external supervisor.

I was writing a thesis on chronic pain management and the impact of imagery and stretch-based relaxation on an outpatient population. I was challenging a research base that was conducted at Duke University in North Carolina where they carried out this experiment with admitted patients. I was proving that it would work on an outpatient basis too so there was a lot of clinical work needed.

However, I had actually conducted all of my field research, done the interviews, used the questionnaires and performed the techniques with the patients. Since I only needed to finish the write-up, I could do without her. Rather than telling her I was withdrawing her as my external supervisor, I thought it was best to just leave it as it was without her responding.

I omitted telling her because I knew I was actually moving to the University of Sussex to work with Mic Cooper (now Professor Mic Cooper) and the late Dr Mick Burton.

So I knew I wouldn't be in this unseen, horrible battle for much longer. However, if I had known now what you're reading about narcissism and codependency, it would have helped me so much because I still thought that I was bad. I felt alone and under constant threat for nearly two years.

I tried to box it and did exceedingly well, missing out on a first by three points while doing several jobs, being a dad and fighting this war at the hospital that nobody else knew was going on apart from her and me.

When I got to Sussex University, I bought a house in Brighton and was trying to settle with my daughter.

I was starting my Master's degree in Counselling Psychology and was working at the hospital in Brighton (both in the Morley Street young adults' centre and as the mental health practitioner for the health centre).

Then one day, Mick Burton called me into his office and said, "I need to see you as a matter of urgency." He sat me down and said, "Now don't worry too much but we've got some concerns. Your reference from (this consultant psychologist) states that you have an issue with power."

Everything was suddenly on the line.

I told him, very economically, what was going on and explained that he could check with my internal supervisor whom I had as a confidante. I asked him if I could please stay on my Master's degree and keep my positions.

For those two years, I had to really make myself small because I thought that if I asserted myself in any way, they were going to think she was right about my issue with power. So her damage to me continued over a four year span. When I finished my dissertation thesis, Professor Mic Cooper said, "You're not very confident in what you do but you've done a brilliant job; this is excellent work." Even today, that thesis is still being taken out of Sussex University and used as reference work.

Yet I had no confidence because of the battering I had got and that one remark. Why would somebody do that? Why would they want to continue the attack?

And it's this. A narcissist isn't done with you until they say they are!

CHAPTER 9

NARCISSISM & CODEPENDENCY IN BUSINESS PARTNERSHIPS

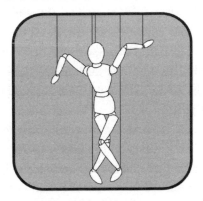

*"Leave once, they're the fool. Leave twice, you're the fool:
Get out of Dodge!"*
-Michael Padraig Acton-

BEWARE THE CAREER NARCISSIST AND SIGNING UNHEALTHY BUSINESS AGREEMENTS: A warning message for shareholders, business partners and employees By Marty Davis, Attorney, Business Consultant and Managing Partner, LegalSolutionsGrp.com

Are you someone looking to set up or transform a business or embark on a new partnership? Understanding codependent and narcissistic traits—in self and others—will help you to avoid poisonous partnerships and build great teams.

Much of my work involves business development and creating new business entities, including business protection.

However, I also become involved in existing business relationships that have become sour and that need to navigate a change of direction. With modified agreements or effective legal mediation, when they are heading towards a bitter ending, 'business' really can avoid economic catastrophe.

To avoid getting into the latter situation, we should always be mindful of the balance of responsibilities among partners. As Shaw Family Law reminds us: codependency describes a relationship where one partner sacrifices his or her own needs to fulfil the other's.

In an unequal partnership, you could find yourself taking on the brunt of the responsibility for driving success leading to overwork, perfectionism and internalised shame if things don't work out. As a result of this type of brutal culture, burnout often cripples people and company success along with it. A narcissistic partner may reap the rewards of your hard labour but keep you in your place by shaming you, belittling your accomplishments and creating chaos so that whatever goal you are set to reach, the objective is moved just before you can cement (and claim) your achievement.

One of the first signs of codependency creeping into a business is often one partner taking on an uneven share of the workload. As the other partner/s pull back on the time, effort, and care they are giving to the business, the codependent partner instinctively fills the gap by working harder. As soon as this happens, the relationship has already started shifting in an unhealthy direction.

The importance of personality attributes for team success
People are the greatest determining factor of success in business.

It's their creativity, motivation style, drive, management style and people skills that determine success.

So, in creating or transforming an enterprise, who you go into business with and why are vitally important. It doesn't matter whether it's a corporation or a partnership but having a shared vision and clearly defined steps to reach your goals are key.

Intrinsic to that is determining the roles of the shareholders, which in turn relates back to individual personalities.

If a business proposition seems too good to be true. . . you guessed it. It probably is. Narcissists build up a person, charm a board of directors and convince businesses they can deliver wealth and success. They then quickly, smoothly and cunningly move in to control, manipulate and take.

Remember, from what Michael Padraig Acton has stated clearly in this book, a narcissist is only done with you when they are done. They may initially offer collateral, blood and promises but like a tick, leech or Count Dracula, their real aim is always to self-serve, without remorse and suck you dry.

Most leaders have narcissistic traits, but are these traits likely to hamper the success of the organisation or partnership? Will they affect the hiring practices of the business? Are they going to change the culture of the organisation? The culture of a business needs to be driven but when does this become excessive and toxic for employees and business partners?

Business is about making money but businesses also depend upon employees' wellbeing, productivity, kindness and willingness to please.

The following account was chosen from an interview with an employee who works in a severely toxic business culture.

This employee was chosen to specifically illustrate what can happen in such a scenario.

Narcissist at the helm: a case study

I work for a fairly small, private software company of just under 200 people. It was a family-owned company run by a very dynamic, personable CEO but he passed away several years ago before I started and they brought in this new CEO.

He has been in start-ups and turned them over multiple times so he wanted to turn us into this Silicon Valley type success story, bring in a new team and change the culture.

I think the whole organisation is now full of narcissists but one person in particular has really been problematic and, for me personally, probably the most difficult person I've ever had to work with. He has put me through a wide range of emotions.

First impressions: entitled and antagonistic

I met him in my first onsite interview, which was actually his first day at the company. The position for which I was being interviewed was not in my preferred field because I didn't have the experience to qualify for much above an entry level position. I was therefore returning to a field in which I had previous experience.

I felt vulnerable explaining that in the interview but he kept coming back to that point saying things like, 'Why would you make a change now?' It felt a little bit humiliating.

He kept poking and digging and almost making me repeat what had happened.

Even the Vice President said, "She already explained why she's in the job market. Do you think we can move on?"

He asked me about culture and how I felt about working with different cultures. He pointed out that I was a white American and I felt that was a little bit inappropriate for an interview, at least the way that he phrased it. I answered it as diplomatically as I could because I have worked in international companies and have a lot of experience working with people from all over; I enjoy it.

He came across like he was just trying to cut me down and put me in my place. Here he was, on his first day and I felt like I was on the defensive which I've never felt before in an interview. I've always felt that interviews were an opportunity for mutual discovery but he was just very antagonistic. That was my first impression.

Aloof from the crowd

One of the changes that he's put into place is that you don't deal with him directly anymore. He's put in layers of management so things have to move up this ladder. He's been bringing in a lot of really young kids who just follow him and do whatever he says without question. You just don't bother him unless it's gone through this chain of command. It's very strange.

He's very big on PR. There's a real focus on how he is perceived and how the company is perceived.

He's trying to paint this picture but underneath the company is a mess. Then there was the whole thing with his appearance. There's being well-dressed and well-groomed but he always looks unreal. There's nothing out of place.

Everything is very controlled and coordinated to the nth degree.

A lack of empathy emerges

Right after he started, there were some lay-offs. He referred to the people who had been laid off as 'the departed' like they were deceased or something. He sent an email to the entire company and the tone was rather disparaging towards those people. Many of them had been with the company for a very long time so it was a sensitive area. The email contained images and one of them showed figures standing, saluting someone. I guess he was supposed to be the person in the middle with a circle of people around him saluting him in a military or almost Hitler-esque way. It was very strange.

There was another image of a figure holding someone who was slumped down. It said something like, 'Sometimes, some must fall before the others can move on.'

I asked myself, "Where am I?" I felt that was a lack of empathy towards the people who had been let go and those who had worked with them.

I had a bad experience with him a couple of months after I had started. I had to work from home because I was unable to drive for a couple of weeks following surgery.

By this time, he had cut a lot of policies that the company had had in place for a long time. One of the biggest was remote work arrangements, a really big thing in this area because some people commute long distances.

So he really wanted me to try and get to work any way that I could. I didn't want to make waves because I was so new to the role so I took the train to work one day.

It's really not a good train system here so it took me about three hours to get to and from work that day. I wasn't able to drive yet.

I told him, "I tried to take the train today but I was in pain and exhausted. I need some more time before I can drive to work again. I need to be remote a little more." He basically just said that that wasn't acceptable so I ended up going to HR and they told me to get a note from my doctor and not discuss it with him, basically.

I discussed this with my therapist and she said, "You never should have tried to go to work. Your doctor said you're not supposed to be in a car. What were you thinking taking the train?"

I said, "I don't know" and that's one of the feelings I get from my experiences with him. I would do things that I knew I shouldn't be doing or that were harmful to me to try and please him. I know better but then I just do it anyway and then I feel terrible and unhappy with myself afterwards.

A narcissistic rage

While I was working from home, he called me a lot, almost like he was checking up with me.

I had to have a couple of meetings with him and they were very contentious because he wanted me to do something in a way that really didn't make sense. I was explaining to him the way it should be done, based on my experience, because I'm the expert in that area. He got very, very angry with me for going against him. I pushed it a little bit.

I was respectful but I said, "Why am I here? Why was I hired to do this if you don't want to listen to the best way to do it based on my experience?"

He got very, very upset and dismissive and kept saying, "Are we done here?" and started doing other things on his computer.

But he continued to call me and hit me up on Skype all the time just for nothing, just kind of pestering me.

No genuine praise; no remorse

He can never just say, "You did a great job!"

He would say things like, "I really like the work you've been doing on this newsletter but was really hoping that you would have done this, there were some typos that I had to fix, etc," you know? I've seen him do this to others also.

He has mentioned that really contentious meeting we had while I was working remotely but not to apologise.

He says things such as, "You were really upset with me in those days. I'm glad that we're much better now."

That stuck out to me when I read through this book. I understood, "Oh, that is exactly something that a narcissist would do: try to put it back on me and make it my fault or make it seem like it was something else."

Surviving the corporate narcissist

I've really had to work on my boundaries. For example, in my phone navigation app, I have relabelled the office address as, 'Time Limited Destination' so I am reminded every day that it's not forever.

I also have a little thing on my desk that says something to the effect of, "let it go." If it's not going to affect me in the long-term then I just need to let it go, not dwell on it and move on.

I don't really want to get too involved with anyone on a friendship level at work. First of all, because there are a lot of people trying to please him and it's hard to know who to trust. But also, a lot of it is because I've drawn this boundary over how much I'll give. Every once in a while, I go over it and regret it but I have a very definite boundary in my mind. I don't interact with people from my company on LinkedIn or anything. I've tried to downplay my professional link with them. I try to put work in a box.

Since I don't feel like I always accomplish a lot there, I've had to find other things to put my energy into. Sometimes it's cooking or making something. I've found that those kinds of things help since I am holding back at work. Work does come up a lot in my own personal therapy. We have talked about how to manage it. I guess that would be another tip. If you are going to stay in a company like this or work for someone like this you are going to need to talk to someone about it. You are going to need to have reminders and a plan on how to manage it.

Learning lessons: the mark of the career narcissist
If a narcissist is put into a position of power, as with the situation above, you will almost certainly notice a hit to your employees' performances and a reduction in their overall wellbeing. It would be a very good idea for you to not only consider your own plight, in terms of your business agreement, but to also listen to your employees. After all, the person profiled here could very easily gather evidence and sue the company or even press charges.

If you are in a business partnership with a narcissist, you are likely to find that your partner continually makes you out to be the problem. "Why are you complaining when we are doing so well?" "It's your constant issues that are bringing our company down?"

Sound familiar?

In either case, the corporate leader or business partner wielding NPD-type control may not be aware they are doing anything wrong. They will probably conduct all aspects of their life in the same way.

Resolving a bad business arrangement

How does one avoid getting into this situation? If the business is successful but things are not completely on your terms, how can you turn things around to create a win-win outcome? How are adverse issues best handled?

First, check your forming documents, where written. Do they give you any guidance on a way forward?

Second, could you use the strengths of one partner to shore up the shortcomings of another? It might even be prudent for you to make use of a mediator because in my experience, sometimes partners or shareholders are too close to the issues to be able to step back and create a workable solution.

Ultimately though, the law will have set in stone most aspects of a signed agreement. This is why a legal consult needs to be your first stepping stone to returning to business safety.

Although Michael Padraig Acton could help you to identify and plan to exit a toxic personal relationship, business and employee agreements are different. There are many specific issues and hurdles that need to be managed, navigated and overcome. If you are already in a mess then I strongly advise you to seek legal guidance before you do anything else.

My closing advice, whether you are with a toxic business partner or you are an employee in a toxic company, is to take some safe steps to clarify what the issues are and your ideal resolution.

Your suffering has to end and you will need appropriate legal and personal support to help you come to a healthy conclusion. The part of my legal work I love most is helping people identify their issues (as they are not always clear), working with those issues to find a path to resolution and helping to free them from the fear of change so they can act with confidence.

Again, I cannot reiterate enough how essential it is you receive expert legal guidance. Law is not about empathy or compassion, it is about agreements and protection. If you are not a lawyer then you need guidance from one as soon as possible. Many times, in my practice as a business lawyer I have been asked, too late, to fix everything. Don't make the same mistake!

RECOMMENDED READING

Do you Work for a Narcissistic Organisation? —https://www.
psychologytoday.com/us/blog/your-personal-renaissance/201804/
do-you-work-narcissistic-organization

How to Work for a Narcissistic Boss—https://hbr.org/2016/04/
how-to-work-for-a-narcissistic-boss

Narcissistic Leaders: The Incredible Pros, the Inevitable Cons—
https://hbr.org/2004/01/narcissistic-leaders-the-incredible-
pros-the-inevitable-cons

*How Does Leader Narcissism Influence Employee Voice: The
Attribution of Leader Impression Management and Leader-Member
Exchange*—https://www.ncbi.nlm.nih.gov/pmc/articles/PMC6571719/

*Narcissistic Leadership: How to Identify Narcissists and Cope
with Narcissism at Work*—https://www.ckju.net/en/blog/
narcissistic-leadership-how-identify-narcissists-and-cope-
narcissism-work/31265

Detaching Yourself from a Codependent Relationship—https://
www.kanecountydivorceattorneys.com/st-charles-lawyers/
codependent-relationship

CHAPTER 10

AVOIDING DOMESTIC VIOLENCE: TRACKING, TRACING AND STOPPING THE NARCISSIST

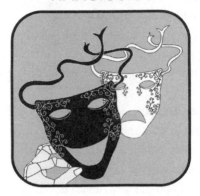

"Hurt souls: harder to think love is safe."
-Michael Padraig Acton-

If domestic abuse at the hands of a narcissist stopped at one person, it would be bad enough. But the damage perpetrated by Narcissistic Personality Disorder spreads like a wildfire.

That is why part of my work is dedicated to finding a lasting solution to the silent pandemic of NPD abuse that is spreading disaster and, yes, and often death across the world.

I have mentioned many times that the narcissist sucks their victim dry and then moves on to another host. Since they never learn from their mistakes and are rarely brought to justice, the cycle continues.

To me, the key lies in strengthening the connection between NPD and domestic violence. Domestic violence is an issue which has seen enormous progress over recent years and this protects people because it has been criminalised.

But first, let's look at how closely NPD abuse maps on to domestic violence.

What does NPD abuse look like?

Codependents in a relationship with a narcissist can expect to be routinely humiliated, isolated, controlled and accused of being and doing wrong. A narcissist will humiliate you by:

- Shouting and screaming at you.
- Swearing at you and calling you names.
- Constantly putting you down and criticising your intelligence, sanity, capability, looks and other qualities.
- Claiming you are worthless, undesirable and beneath them.
- Comparing you (negatively) with others.
- Embarrassing you in front of others.
- Downplaying your achievements (often claiming the credit for any success you have enjoyed).
- Dismissing or ridiculing your interests.
- Using sarcasm to hurt you and then claiming you're 'too sensitive' to take their 'jokes.'
- Winding you up until you react.

Returning to our earlier case study, with Jackie and John, we can see some real examples of this abusive behaviour in action.

On a train journey, Jackie was very excited about a change in her college course. She had chosen a better schedule and was sharing the details with John. Within two seconds, Jackie was crushed. John dismissed what she was saying, in a very polite and charming way but so that it demeaned her achievement. He told her he had bigger fish to fry and things going on that she doesn't even know about. He's pleased for her but why ruin the evening by reminding him of his own hectic schedule.

On another occasion, Jackie wanted to go to her favourite restaurant. At first, John seemed happy and agreed they would go there. Then, all of a sudden, he was criticising the cost of things and asking Jackie, 'How are we going to afford this?', 'Don't you think this is extravagant?' and 'Why are you putting this on me and always draining me of money?' So not only did he ruin the evening but Jackie felt terrible for even suggesting the meal out. Be mindful, it was her birthday.

A narcissist will isolate you by:

- Stopping you from having hobbies or socialising without them.
- Controlling your movements and activities.
- Trying to stop you from seeing family and friends.
- Turning others against you (often claiming you're unstable).
- Withholding affection or abandoning you and then claiming you're too needy.
- Ignoring your feelings.
- Pretending they know better than you how you feel.
- Downplaying your problems.
- Pretending others share their negative opinion of you.

One way a narcissist might stop a codependent from seeing friends and family members is to sabotage their enjoyment.

Jackie was planning to see her mum in Germany. She had bought gifts for the trip the night before and was very excited about going.

Then, all of a sudden, John stopped communicating with her and became very stoic. He said he could no longer take her to the airport because something important had come up at work. In fact, she was leaving at the worst time possible.

This was manipulation designed to ruin Jackie's enjoyment of the trip and leave her feeling unsupported and isolated.

A narcissist will control you by:

- Making you do things you don't want to do (this includes pressurising or forcing you into having sex).
- Threatening to harm (or kill) you or those you love.
- Claiming your children are at risk of being taken into care.
- Threatening to commit suicide if you leave.
- Preventing you from leaving the house.
- Denying you access to money, your car or your phone.
- Damaging your property.
- Tracking your calls, emails and search history.
- Following and constantly calling you.
- Making decisions on your behalf.
- Ordering you around.
- Being overly temperamental (forcing you to 'walk on eggshells').

- Stopping you from accessing medical help.
- Claiming you will always be theirs and they will always track you down.

It is important to note that with NPD, domestic violence is rarely physical. Any physical abuse is usually concealed carefully to keep up the façade of the perfect relationship and, for the benefit of everyone else, a perfect persona.

Control is usually exerted by emotional manipulation and financial abuse, etc.

A narcissist will accuse you of:

- Having love affairs or flirting.
- Making them abuse you.
- Being the reason for their problems.
- Being mistaken about things you know are true (gaslighting).
- Being ungrateful for their efforts.
- Getting upset over nothing.
- Taking their jokes too seriously.
- Abusing them!

After spending time in a relationship with a narcissist, you will find your own character changing. You might start:

- Prioritising their needs over yours.
- Blaming yourself for their behaviour.
- Downplaying or making excuses for their behaviour (to yourself and others).

- Changing plans to avoid upsetting them or because they make you feel guilty.
- Bottling up your feelings.
- Feeling numb or hopeless.
- Feeling guilty for speaking your mind.
- Giving up things to make them happy.
- Worrying what will happen if you leave them.
- Sharing their criticisms of you.

These are the very same tactics used in domestic violence; now a punishable offence in over 120 countries following amazing global campaigning activity throughout the 21st century.

Where are we with domestic violence?
In 2013, the UK's definition of domestic violence changed. For the first time, coercive control was accepted as part of the picture and the definition was extended to include domestic abuse, making it clear that the damage to victims goes beyond physical violence.

This was an important step forward because people with NPD are usually too cunning to leave visible signs of their abuse.

The full definition of domestic violence and abuse in the UK is (in 2021):

Any incident or pattern of incidents of controlling, coercive or threatening behaviour, violence or abuse between those aged 16 or over who are or have been intimate partners or family members regardless of gender or sexuality.

This can encompass, but is not limited to, the following types of abuse:

- Psychological
- Physical
- Sexual
- Financial
- Emotional

Controlling behaviour is: a range of acts designed to make a person subordinate and/or dependent by isolating them from sources of support, exploiting their resources and capacities for personal gain, depriving them of the means needed for independence, resistance and escape and regulating their everyday behaviour.

Coercive behaviour is: an act or a pattern of acts of assault, threats, humiliation and intimidation or other abuse that is used to harm, punish, or frighten their victim.

This definition recognises the role of isolation and the overall context of power and control. You will notice how perfectly this definition maps on to the pattern of behaviours used by narcissists to control their victims.

In the US, domestic violence is defined in relation to state domestic violence laws, as follows:

Felony or misdemeanour crimes of violence committed by a current or former spouse or intimate partner of the victim, by a person with whom the victim shares a child in common, by a person who is cohabitating with or has cohabitated with the victim as a spouse or intimate partner, by a person similarly situated to a spouse of the victim under the domestic or family violence laws of the jurisdiction receiving grant monies, or by any other person against an adult or youth victim who is protected from that person's acts under the domestic or family violence laws of the jurisdiction.

In the US, domestic violence definitions and how crimes are coded in the state legislature varies by state (e.g. some states recognise dating relationships more explicitly than others). However, none of these definitions make any connection between domestic violence and narcissistic personality disorder.

Whether working at federal/country or state/county level, there needs to be a way of making this NPD label stick. This will be a positive move both in terms of victim support and when domestic abuse cases are filed in a court of law. So that when a narcissist is caught, they are made to pay for the mental and emotional hurt they have caused. Too often they slip through the net, brush themselves down and go in search of another person to feed off of leaving the victim wrung out, scared, depleted and sometimes dead.

An important note on teenage relationship abuse

While domestic violence affects people of all ages, genders, ethnic groups, social classes and sexualities, it is recognised, in both the UK and US that teenagers are particularly vulnerable.

According to the UK government, teens are more likely to accept abusive and violent behaviour than older people. This was based on a 2009 research project carried out in schools by the National Society for the Prevention of Cruelty to Children

(NSPCC) and backed up by figures from the 2011/12 Crime Survey for England and Wales.

The NSPCC report also revealed that teens often felt that adults trivialised their experiences of domestic abuse and that they were more likely to confide in friends than parents or professionals.

Added to this is the age barrier, which prevents under-18s from accessing some support services for victims of abuse.

In response, separate definitions have now been created under the terms teenager relationship abuse (TRA), in the UK, and teen dating violence (TDV) in the US.

Although there has been much progress made in recognising non-physical domestic violence (especially by males against female partners), a diagnosis of NPD does not currently carry any weight in a domestic abuse case. Yet, a relationship with someone with NPD will always become a toxic, abusive relationship. The narcissist knows no other way to behave and does not change.

Joining the dots
Joined-up working between psychologists, psychiatrists, social services, lawyers/attorneys and judges is the key to linking domestic violence and NPD abuse—a similar team in fact to that involved in developing this book.

Imagine:

- If psychologists experienced in working with NPD were routinely recruited as expert witnesses.
- If the legal system recognised that NPD abuse and domestic abuse are one and the same.

- If social services were able to provide specific NPD abuse support for victims.

Then, we might finally see more restrictions on a narcissist's ability to do harm. How could this happen on the ground, what would it look like?

Here are some practical suggestions and what I am working towards developing:

- The establishment of recognised NPD abuse specialist law practices. Psychologists could then appropriately refer victims seeking legal help.
- Creation of a database of NPD abuse expert witnesses.
- Change in law to recognise NPD abuse as a specific form of domestic violence. This would help to inform interventions for adult and teenage perpetrators.
- Recruitment of NPD abuse advisors. In the UK, we already have Independent Domestic Violence Advisers (IDVAs) working with victims. If independent NPD abuse advisers were also available to support victims of diagnosed narcissists, outcomes could be improved.
- Representation on safeguarding boards, domestic violence forums and multi-agency risk assessment conferences (MARACs)*.
- For teen victims in the UK, NPD abuse advisers and lawyers could be represented on Local Safeguarding Children Boards (LSCBs). This would help strengthen the safety net at a local level and nip the problem at its bud.
- Strengthening of care pathways linking all of the above elements.

- Specific NPD abuse training for social workers, health professionals, youth offending teams, magistrates, police officers and legal prosecutors.
- Creation of NPD abuse tools/resources for display on the websites of relevant domestic violence, health and justice organisations.

*MARACs have already been proven to reduce revictimisation in domestic violence cases.

I would be happy to work with government agencies, NGOs, legal practices, the justice system and medical professionals to help create such a strong NPD/domestic violence pathway and reduce the harm being done in society by these uncontrolled monsters. This really is about educating the public and professional bodies of how to identify NPD and how to manage, log and act upon the destruction they leave behind.

The elusive narcissist: a warning from Oliver Twist
I wanted to finish this section with an example from popular, classic literature. While researching this chapter, I realised that the subtle distinction between domestic violence and NPD abuse is cleverly referenced in that Charles Dickens favourite, Oliver Twist.

If I were to ask you who the domestic abuser is in Oliver Twist, the character Bill Sikes would immediately spring to mind. He is the classic 'wife beater' who ends up with Nancy's blood on his hands. From that moment on, his days are numbered.

But I leave you to reflect on the character of Edward Leeford aka Monks. His mind twisted by his own mother, Leeford feels so entitled to Oliver's inheritance that he has no qualms in hunting down and destroying his innocent half-brother. He does this through lies and deceit, paying Fagin to corrupt Oliver and destroying any evidence linking Oliver to his mother.

Sarah Phelps' version of Monks, in her 2007 miniseries, is even more the classic narcissist. Now a handsome and cultured gentleman, he charms and gaslights his grandfather Mr Brownlow and seeks to seduce and abuse the attractive Rose Maylie through a combination of isolation and coercive control.

While Phelps gives a touch of humanity to Sikes (who loves his dog) and Fagin (who shows some concern for Oliver), the entitled Monks is portrayed as totally without remorse.

And while Dickens' Monks does eventually end up in jail, the fate of Phelps' character is unclear. We only know that he is sent away to the West Indies, free to devise his next Machiavellian scheme—and without a speck of blood on his well-manicured hands!

It may seem unusual for a psychologist to advocate for criminalising a psychiatric disorder but this is not about punishment—it is about tracking, tracing and neutralising a very real psychological plague. It is also about educating people so that NPD abuse is more visible and therefore people are more protected.

CHAPTER 11

A MEETING OF MINDS

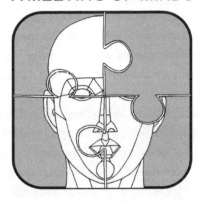

"Part of my work is dedicated to finding a lasting solution to the silent pandemic of NPD abuse."
-Michael Padraig Acton-

JOINING THE DOTS OF DOMESTIC VIOLENCE AND NARCISSISTIC PERSONALITY DISORDER: A MEETING OF MINDS
By Susan Weitzman and Michael Padraig Acton

Coming out of lockdown, domestic violence is so topical at the time of writing that we need to tackle the issue head on. I was pleased that we had included the previous chapter on domestic violence but I wasn't satisfied—it needed something more.

Then, as the book was just about to go to print, I had a response from an email I had sent three months earlier. It was from Susan Weitzman. My whole life has been synchronicity-synchrodestiny led. Another reinforcement to the metaphysical laws we little understand. Due to the pandemic, Susan and her husband, psychologist Richard Goldwasser, have been involved with remote schooling their three children via Zoom, as well as maintaining their busy clinical practices, serving people especially stressed during these pandemic times. She had been meaning to get back to my email for months. It was a real 'hold the press' moment, of course, and I quickly arranged for us to have a chat. And what a chat it was.

Susan is the author of *Not to People Like Us: Hidden Abuse in Upscale Marriages*, a book that was so topical it garnered an enormous amount of interest both in the US and abroad. She has appeared on countless TV shows including Oprah, 20/20 and The Today Show, and is also a researcher and clinical psychotherapist who helps victims of domestic violence, predominantly women, to escape their situation. The Founder and President of The Weitzman Center, her many years of work and research led to her uncovering a heretofore unnamed and unresearched phenomenon, which she has called "Upscale Violence."

Susan's work has influenced popular culture including the television series Big Little Lies (for which she received credit by author Liane Moriarty) as well as the movie Girl on the Train (Paula Hawkins). As an expert witness, she has participated in some high-profile criminal cases around the world. She is a sought-after consultant and expert witness, a clinician who is both empathic and insightful in her work.

What follows is the result of this meeting of minds where we discovered we shared so much, including a style of talking straight. Like myself, Susan uses strong, real-life examples and what she terms "buzz phrases" to communicate her insights so that the reader or listener can understand what she is communicating.

For example, she refers to the concept of "slot machine love" in her book to explain why battered men and women stay for so long in abusive relationships. Ironically, our synchronicity emerged, as this is an expression I so often use, too. As Susan so eloquently puts it, regarding our connection, "we are often looking at the same river but from different sides." She goes on to say, "People who stay in torturous relationships are waiting for the jackpot, as it may have paid off early on. Sadly, the payoff is unpredictable and unreliable." I believe that the payoff is not going to come. They invest and invest and invest and they wonder, should they pull out or keep trying to win the big one?

Breaking the mould

Susan's book, 'Not to People Like Us' and the publicity afterwards saved many lives. "I have had women say, 'When you were on Nightline 20/20, that's when I left my marriage. That TV show episode helped me to leave.' Or an outpouring of letters about how 'relieving and freeing' it was to know that what they were experiencing did exist, even to people like us."

Susan shared with me an origin story of her research. "I was teaching at the University of Chicago when conducting my research about this population. In one of my most popular classes, I said I was conducting research on domestic violence among an upscale population and asked if anyone knew of any women who had experienced this, who I could speak to privately. In the first or second class, a guy walks into the room, papers flying. He looked like Columbo, seemingly disorganised.

"He turned out to be one of the biggest divorce attorneys in Chicago and told me he could get me a whole compilation of cases because that was the population he was dealing with. He had his secretary call all of these women and asked them to speak to me because these women didn't easily come forward; they were embarrassed and so in some ways seeking them out was like searching for unicorns.

"That population was unique to my study and my book." Susan's years of research continued and the resulting work actually broke the mould. No one had studied this before.

"If you read the first page of my book, it's a true vignette with the names adjusted to protect the identity of the innocent. In the anecdote, the woman threw a surprise party for her husband and at the end of the party she gave the guests cake to take home. He proceeded to beat her up because he liked the cake and 'how dare she do that!'

"A lot of the abuse is emotional which, sometimes, is far worse in some ways because the physical wounds will heal but the emotional scars stay a long time.

"Here's what happens with narcissists in these relationships. They go for the vulnerable victim because they can smell blood in the water. Then, it's like boiling a frog where the water just gets hotter and hotter over time.

"They convince their victims that they're worthless. What they share is that they both have a low image of her. In the book, I speak about a brilliant woman with a PhD. Her husband told her, 'When I divorce you, I'm going to fight you in court so you will be penniless, selling pencils on the street.' She believed him because of the gradual decimation of her self-esteem."

"The veil of silence"

"People would sometimes say to me, 'Why are your women different?' (somehow, they became *my* women). I would say, that's not the point! This is about inclusivity not exclusivity. Until this research, these women were living under what I call a *'veil of silence'* as they were not typically seen as victims of domestic abuse. In part, it is because they don't fit the stereotype, but often, it is because they have nowhere to easily seek out help.

"It's about different demographics. Often, when low socio-economic women come out about domestic abuse, they are believed immediately. They can fit straight into the shelter environment. Upscale women can't go to shelters, as they seem so different and are made to feel so. They go to court and no one believes them. They are excluded. Oftentimes, they are married to very powerful men who are either beloved and respected or are paying for their wife's relatives or friends in various ways. They don't want to cut off the golden cow. Instead of coming out, there's a self-inflicted veil of silence. Usually, the abuser isolates the woman from her support source but in upscale marriages the women do it to themselves because they're so embarrassed.

"It's like the husband has her on remote control. Who would believe her? She's not going to tell people at the school or the women she lunches with. Someone wearing a fur who says her husband beat her up before they got on the private jet—who the heck's going to have any pity for them?

"I worked with a well-known professional couple while I was on staff at the Department of Psychiatry at the University of Chicago. I saw them both briefly about communication issues but she returned when she became pregnant. Pregnancy is often a trigger because the narcissist knows he is going to lose the wife's focus and attention. It turns out that she had been hiding that her husband had a torture chamber in the basement. It could only be opened from the outside and he would chain her up. Not like *50 Shades of Gray* but literally torturing her by locking her up with no water and no phone.

"There is also a myth that upscale women have access to money. As I explain in an article featured on www. theweitzmancenter.org, a woman may be living in an affluent household, but she often has as little access to finances as someone with no money at all. We couldn't get funding for my not-for-profit for so long because people assumed these people did not need assistance; what was not realised was that these women didn't have control over the purse strings.

"I've had some well-known people come through my door. Wives of household names where you would never in a million years believe this was going on. I've recently started working as an expert witness on a case where the husband makes US$6 million a year and is inflicting outrageous emotional and financial abuse because his wealth allows him to do so."

A key to healing
"Awareness has to come with external validation for this population because they're so disbelieved and disenfranchised. The families of many of the women I have worked with will

say things like, 'Well, what did you do to get him that angry?' Or, 'He just donated a wing at the hospital and is so beloved. Are you sure of what you are claiming?'

"There are a few buzz phrases that I have coined that really fit the situation. For example, a lot of these women do something I call *justification by explanation*. They'll say, 'Well, he's had a bad day at work.' But that is just a form of denial, going along to get along. However, the water's slowly getting hotter and hotter for the frog until it is too late!

"For many of these women, it's not just about the money. They stay for the kids, the security, and sometimes they stay for the status. They just don't know what else to do.

"I also talk in my book about 'slot machine love.' People stay at the slot machine because every so often it pays off. They call it variable reinforcement. That's why she stays. A lot of women keep thinking about that first date. It was idyllic for years.

"In terms of healing, too often the abused have to hit rock bottom. I do think there has to be an acknowledgement. But what's key, I have learned over many years from this population, is external validation because their self-esteem has been so decimated that they have become terrorised by the narcissist.

"I end my book with a little anecdote about a sculpture I once saw at a craft fair. There was a cage and inside, a little figure was holding on to the bars looking out. What the figure didn't see was that the door behind them was open. I ended my book by saying just as the figure needed to turn around, people need to turn their minds around and they would see that they have the way out."

Getting the message out

Susan has carried out the research for her next book. It is about narcissists in the legal system. We are hoping to collaborate on this venture together.

"This has to come out, what is going on in the courts," she insisted. "Maybe that's why our paths have crossed. Shows like *Big Little Lies* open the door a little but if I had a wish list, *Not to People Like Us* should be a documentary or a movie. It should be out there. The same with the second book. If it was out there, this would change the face of domestic violence."

There has already been mention that the *"Black Widow"* case in this book may be heading for film. It is vital to educate people of this secret that knows no boundaries, genders or sexualities.

I look forward to collaborating with Susan further. It is clear that not enough victims are coming forwards. We only get snippets. We need more money invested into researching the variables of domestic violence and NPD and to discover who's really suffering and how. Suicide is often the result, but this does not address the cause!

I would like to end this chapter by emphasising an important point, which Susan and I share thoughts on. During interviews, I am often asked about what therapists can do to help narcissists themselves. I tell them that narcissists are a very difficult group to treat. Susan tells the women she helps the same, "You think you can fix it because you fix everything else. But these are people who cannot easily be fixed no matter how hard their wives may have tried."

"Relationships with a narcissist are challenging," she says. "It is heartbreaking to say the writing is on the wall. Sometimes, if they don't want to hear it, they leave the therapeutic relationship. But if they stay with therapy, they at least have a chance to get to the other side. I will add that there certainly are researched techniques for working with the narcissistic personality, but there has to be a lot of motivation on that person's part for it to make a difference. It is sadly true that they are a difficult group to treat."

We need to find a way to argue NPD-victim cases in court better, Sarah Zabel's judicial contribution to this book clearly highlights this, but we must find a way to truly measure and criminalise the actions of cold, ruthless and abhorrent NPDs and their actions.

PART III

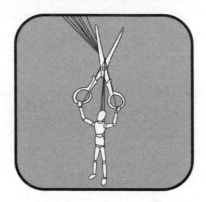

UNHOOKING & RECOVERING FROM A NARCISSIST

CHAPTER 12

BREAKING THE DYNAMIC: HOW DO I QUIT YOU?

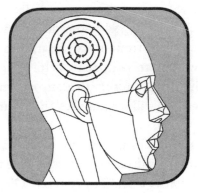

"At first, I was afraid, I was petrified. Kept thinking I could never live without you by my side."
I Will Survive (performed by Gloria Gaynor; written by Freddie Perren/Dino Fekkaris)

Codependency, addiction and self-loathing
Codependency can be partly understood as a disease of self-loathing. I see all the time in my work that by focusing all of their being on serving other people, codependents deny themselves the full light of awareness. They try to nourish themselves from the reflected light of other people's appreciation and gratitude but the presence of self-hate, lurking in the background, leads to a constant, gnawing self-doubt. They sometimes see their own self-disgust lurking behind the smiles of those they are attempting to please and they obsessively work harder to be a better partner, employee, child or parent.

This attachment to another person is an addiction every bit as damaging as an attachment to a substance or behaviour—in fact it can be more so, since the narcissist actively works to become a more irresistible fix.

Having worked in drug dependency units for many years, I can confirm that working with someone who is codependent and unhooking them from a toxic relationship is 10 times more difficult and stressful than helping someone off a highly addictive drug. I'm sure that anyone who works with a similar population will scream, 'Yes' in agreement with this statement.

The very same mechanism that is at work in a substance abuser lurks within a codependent. It is the voice that convinces the self that, 'It will be OK', 'Why change?' 'Oh, just one more last one,' 'It's not that bad,' 'No one knows them like I do,' etc.

What is worse for a codependent is that when they explode, scream for recognition, run away or plead, they are reinforcing their own fears of inadequacy and the thoughts and beliefs they hold about being a bad person.

The hole they dig for themselves in this unhealthy addiction is so deep that no one can convince them until they themselves have had a glimpse that this is not working. This can be after years of being hooked or within the first few months or weeks.

Yes, it is possible for a codependent to be hooked within weeks: the extreme charm, praise and adoration shown by the narcissist—the dance that coaches and reels them in—is so real it seems to be exactly the fix the codependent needs in their life.

The intoxicating feeling that, 'Everything is good in my life now', and that, 'This was the moment he or she arrived to fix it all', is so strong and overwhelmingly 'right' that the codependent strives to recreate that 'hit' throughout their upcoming battle with neglect, invisibility, abuse and degradation.

Addiction and the DSM-5

As I've explained, codependency is not, at this time, officially recognised as an addiction but that does not mean that we can't look to the DSM-5 for information and guidance. It must be realised that diagnoses in psychiatry are permanently in a state of debate and new editions of the DSM will reflect current academic opinion.

For example, the DSM-5 has eradicated separate substance abuse and dependency diagnoses and adopted an addiction scale that runs from mild to severe, explaining the decision as follows:

'In DSM-IV, the distinction between abuse and dependence was based on the concept of abuse as a mild or early phase and dependence as the more severe manifestation. In practice, the abuse criteria were sometimes quite severe.

'The revised substance use disorder, a single diagnosis, will better match the symptoms that patients experience.'

At the same time, the manual casts its net wider and now includes gambling, with internet gaming added to Section III with the following caveat:

'Disorders listed there require further research before their consideration as formal disorders. This condition is included to reflect the scientific literature on persistent and recurrent use of Internet games, and a preoccupation with them, can result in clinically significant impairment or distress.'

Perhaps, in time, codependency will be brought into the fold but, until then, codependents (and therapists like me who work with them) can still derive much benefit from the models of addiction used to understand and help those addicted to substances.

Spotting the patterns

It has also become very clear to me, from working on the front line of therapy, there are certain patterns that emerge time after time. However, whenever I work with someone new, I never know how that is going to unfold.

What they bring to me at times is so masked, so hidden under layers and layers of co-habiting themes and stories that there is usually a waiting game to play before I can begin to formulate what happened to this person, and how we are going to help them out of this 'stuckness'.

As I get into the fourth, fifth or eighth session with a codependent the pattern begins to emerge.

This can take time because the original issues codependents come in with are not always about 'being' a codependent but about the symptoms that stem from being a codependent within the claws of a narcissist. In any case, each person requires a slightly different length of time before they feel safe and connected enough to dig with me.

Codependency may look slightly different in terms of the person's story, demographic and their position in the relationship but I can always recognise it when it raises its face.

However, I do think, 'Hmm, let's not be hasty', as I don't want to find something that isn't really there.

It is always a good thing to be reflective, especially when a dual, manipulative dynamic is evolving—as with John and Jackie who are working on how to survive each other and their relationship.

So, my role at this stage is to check out 'stuff'. Yes, I call it stuff. I approach all of this cloudy, confusing, scary space with this soul presenting to me while remaining open enough to see themes develop that can help with our understanding of the root: what is really going on for them and how they got to be in the chair opposite me.

This is the moment when I ask some big questions; questions you, in reading this book, may need to ask yourself or a dear one. Questions like:

- You said that was a deal-breaker yet you're still in the same situation—what keeps you there?
- It is fear that usually keeps us stuck. What does fear look like to you? What are you fearful of?
- What is reality and what is hope for you? How long have things been good, and how long have you been in love with what could be?
- Have you been in this place before and who with? How did you survive that ending?
- What are your thoughts about meeting someone healthy for you in the future?

Exploring these and similar questions will bring to the surface oxymorons, polemic states of being and areas of conflict that usually turn on a big, bright light of recognition for those waist-high in an NPD/codependency relationship.

This is gut-wrenching stuff and often my gut does feel wrenched because we are working with people's inner fears and vulnerabilities.

It is now worth spending some time considering one factor on which escaping from any form of addiction hinges: motivation.

The role of motivation

Motivation is not a quality you either have or don't have: some people tell me they have no motivation, when the reality is that they are motivated—just not enough to put in the effort that's required to change.

So, motivation can be assessed by degree (how much motivation there is) and type (what the source of the motivation is).

For example, a codependent may become aware that their submissive behaviour is setting a poor example to their children and that may be the strongest source of their motivation to change. Alternatively, they may have a strong desire to follow a particular career path and realise that their relationship is holding them back from putting the necessary effort into that goal.

And unfortunately, in difficult circumstances, that motivation can be staying alive and not killing oneself, or curtailing the murder of the narcissist. The 'stuckness' felt by codependents in an NPD relationship can become so hopeless that these extremes are not that uncommon. However, when such deaths do occur, they are reported as 'completed suicide' or 'provoked murder' and rarely is the motivation examined. A much-needed area of research would involve looking at the relationship dynamic and family history of those involved; this could raise awareness and increase focus on the therapeutic and prevention level.

When I reveal to a codependent that motivation is a pliable quality, it provides something to work with. In other words, various therapeutic techniques can be applied to increase the degree of motivation until it is strong enough to effect real change.

The most basic but also the most powerful of these therapeutic tools is to 'mirror' the patient. Through accurate mirroring, much awareness can be elicited which forms the start of the motivation to change. Take this example:

"So he did this last year, you told him that you were worth more than that, and after he did this again last month you are still with him. So you are worth more and still with him?"

Or:

"It has been three years since you held hands or had intimacy and she has continued having affairs. You have compensated by drinking more every night and this works for you?"

Accurate and honest reflecting needs to be carried out in a trusting relationship and my patients need to have reached the position where they feel that what I say, no matter how hard it is for them to hear, is for their good and delivered in a caring and compassionate way. Therapists working in this way visibly see the lightbulbs go on when they get this reflection right and use it at the right time.

It really depends at what stage of development the person is at: it is usual for codependents to go in and out of therapy many times before they get to the stage where they are ready to fully consider the possibility of leaving or changing up their relationship.

This is much the same as a person who is dependent on substances, such as alcohol or drugs, as it can take them several attempts before they are physically and emotionally ready. At times, accurate reflection can be too challenging and the patient will feel that I do not understand them, or they will feel guilty talking about their partner in such a way.

However, every exposure to healthy influences forms part of that necessary withdrawal process. That includes exposure to friends, family, strangers (those witnessing uncomfortable interaction or treatment). It also includes self-realisation and last, but not least, the person's therapist chipping away with, 'This relationship dynamic really does not seem to be good for you'.

Only after withdrawal can the person lock in the motivators that will provide them with the strength to protect their sense of self from the harmful contraindications of this toxic and unhealthy love nest.

So, before motivation must come awareness. Whether a codependent is working with me or trying to help themselves under their own steam, there has to be the recognition that there is a problem and the desire to change. Otherwise there is only a token effort and the entrenched pattern of behaviour will simply keep on repeating itself; as Einstein once put it,

'Insanity (is) doing the same thing over and over again and expecting different results'.

Motivation has to be preceded by awareness of either the harmful effects of the addictive behaviour or the benefits of breaking free—preferably both. This is the starting point of the Stages of Change model that follows in the next chapter.

RECOMMENDED READING

Break Free: Disarm, Defeat, and Beat The Narcissist and Psychopath-Pamela Kole

Escape: How to Beat the Narcissist-H. G. Tudor

Exorcism: Purging the Narcissist from Heart and Soul-H. G. Tudor

Healing from Hidden Abuse: A Journey Through the Stages of Recovery from Psychological Abuse-Shannon Thomas

Healing from a Narcissistic Relationship: A Caretaker's Guide to Recovery, Empowerment, and Transformation-Margalis Fjelstad

The Journey: A Roadmap for Self-Healing After Narcissistic Abuse-Meredith Miller

No Contact With the Narcissist: Escaping Narcissism & Narcissistic Personality Disorder-James Aniston

Run Sis: A Survivor's Guide for Escaping Narcissistic Abuse-Charisma Deberry

Revenge: How to Beat the Narcissist-H. G. Tudor

Whole Again: Healing Your Heart and Rediscovering Your True Self After Toxic Relationships and Emotional Abuse-Jackson MacKenzie

CHAPTER 13

THE UNHOOKING PROCESS

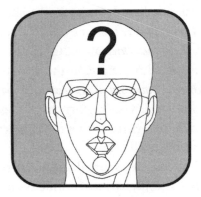

"Even if you have left a narcissist. . . free?"
-Michael Padraig Acton-

Six stages of change
There are several models of addiction, which I could use when working with codependents, but one of the most popular and effective is the Stages of Change Model devised by Professors James Prochaska and Carlo DiClemente in the 1970s. Also referred to as the TTM (Transtheoretical Model), this breaks down the process of addiction recovery into six parts.

I.   **Pre-contemplation**
At the pre-contemplation stage, any recognition of a need to change is mostly unconscious. There may be the occasional flash of awareness when the relationship and health costs of addiction are recognised, but at this stage the benefits provided by the object of addiction, whether a substance, activity or

person, outweigh those costs. In the example of codependency, the security and validity gained from the relationship seem worth the pain. The defining feature of Stage One of the TTM model is the lack of any real motivation to change.

Moreover, it is very rare for someone to access my services at this stage unless they are pushed by a dear one. Even if pushed and sitting with me due to the encouragement of a loved one, nothing, nothing will change until the codependent is ready and, as mentioned before, this can take several attempts, sometimes over several years, before full engagement is made and we can investigate change.

Even then, at this determined stage, the fear of change will be immense and present an enormous challenge. It is a particularly difficult stage for all concerned as there is hope and then no hope; more pain; more affirmation that they cannot survive without their narcissist and fear of being alone forever (for who could want them) etc.

I usually bring aspects of the serenity prayer into this part of the work:

> *Grant me the serenity to accept the things I cannot change,*
> *courage to change the things I can,*
> *and wisdom to know the difference.*

It is important to help the person know that they cannot change their narcissist, they can only change themselves. Until this wisdom sets in, they will continue taking care of their narcissist's requirements, needs and wants, feeding them at the expense of themselves.

They will continue to hope, in vain, that they will get more of the good, intimate, adoring, charming crumbs of affection, recognition and respect.

2. Contemplation

When the desire to break free of addiction emerges, the person has moved on to Stage Two of the TTM. This is an exploratory phase and there may be little motivation to actually put in the work necessary.

The person may lack confidence in their ability to beat their addiction, may waver in their commitment and may think and talk in terms of taking action in 'the future.'

However, they are at least aware of the need to change and open to thinking about the issue.

This part of the process is a fragile one and the person may slip back into Stage One at any time. To move on to Stage Three, they have to reach a point where they accept that the negative effects of their addiction outweigh the benefits. They then have to make that crucial decision to commit to the process of becoming unhooked.

3. Preparation

Having risen to the challenge and accepted responsibility for the change process, the person is now in a position to weigh up their options and decide on a strategy. They might decide to book into a rehab centre or seek a therapist (if they are not already working with one). They may even feel able to handle the journey themselves. Their confidence and commitment levels are likely to be high at this point as they anticipate the benefits of freedom. The quicker they can take action, the more likely they are to make some real progress because, despite their decision to change, it is still possible for them to slip back into the contemplation stage at any time.

4. Action

Change is finally occurring at Stage Four with the person learning new skills and drawing deeper insights about their behaviour along the way. The initial period of action is characterised by enthusiasm as the recovering addict discards old ways of behaving and embraces change. If this early momentum can be sustained for six months, the person has reached the Maintenance stage.

5. Maintenance

By Stage Five, a lot of progress will have been made. The person is not free of their addiction but they have established positive patterns of behaviour, gained more self-control and become aware of high-risk situations.

For codependents, this will involve being conscious of when their narcissistic partner is pushing their buttons and stimulating their need to please.

The next task for the recovering addict is to bring together what they have learned and integrate their new way of being into their lives. Although their addiction is now largely under control, they do need to remain vigilant, as relapse is still a risk.

6. Termination

The person has now successfully created a new self-image, which is no longer defined by the substance, or person, they were once addicted to. Their new, healthier behaviour patterns have become fully integrated in their lives and they are reaping the benefits. The presence of the addictive substance, situation or person no longer tempts them from the path.

Even in this final stage of the TTM, there is a small chance of relapse, perhaps in the event of a significant downturn in circumstances, but that risk is now very low.

In substance abuse, embarking on the road to recovery requires that the drugs or drink are removed from the picture.

The blunt truth is that there has to be a separation for full recovery to happen. Unlike substances, addictive people can change their behaviour to maintain their grip on the addict. For example, what is more compelling to the codependent than the phrase, "But I need you; why am I alone?"

Getting out is the only path to healing

I'm sorry to say that the chance of a positive therapeutic outcome for the narcissist is extremely poor although there are professionals who claim to have had an element of success using various types of therapy. The extent of that element would be interesting to study. There is such a shortage of research in this field and it is this that perpetuates the suffering of those silent codependents. However, positive outcomes are very unlikely since narcissists, by their very nature, usually refuse to accept there is anything wrong with them, and those that do attend therapy tend to leave early on in the process, often believing the therapist to be 'beneath them.'

In all the years I've practiced and been involved in working with NPD, no narcissist has ever engaged and worked through therapy with me, although they have tried. They tend to use the language learned during their short time in therapy against their partner and even against me.

They engage with therapy up to the point of being challenged. Then it is just too much to question their fragile façade any further. Narcissists only usually show up in rooms because their victims invite them in the hope of change. Attitude is a very difficult phenomenon to adjust when the person is unwilling or so scared they are unable to try.

However, there is hope for the codependents who have escaped a narcissist's clutches—but only if they get out. There are no two ways about it: a narcissist's victim cannot heal if they remain part of the toxic dynamic in the same way as a wound will not heal around a foreign object.

As soon as the codependent begins to assert their own existence within the relationship, the narcissist will immediately step up their efforts to quell the rebellion—and they will win.

Having read this far, you may be convinced that your partner, work colleague, parent or adult child are narcissistic. . . or you may still have your doubts.

If you are reading this because you are concerned about a significant other suffering from being in a relationship with a narcissist then it is very important that you tread carefully. An NPD is expertly skilled at isolating their victim, so if the narcissistic person gets wind that you are 'interfering,' chances are that they will spin a web that separates you from them too.

Whether you identify as a codependent or not, understand that behaviours that attempt to humiliate, isolate, control or abuse are unacceptable and the sooner you stand up to your abuser and seek help, the shorter your road to healing and happiness will be. As always, we are only able to change our own attitudes and behaviour. You will soon realise whether these efforts are rewarded with the respect they deserve or are incompatible with your relationship.

What next if you realise you need help?
If you have been living as a codependent for your entire life, having the spotlight turned on you and your needs can be uncomfortable and even overwhelming at first. Without somebody to serve and provide for, the emptiness and insecurity inside becomes revealed. For support, I advise you seek help, read a lot, and talk online with other victims. There will be a huge void to fill. Looking after the chaos of an NPD fills our time and world!

If you do seek to work with a therapist, you should make certain that the professional you choose has a proven background in relationship work. It is a tough job helping a person who is very damaged and carefully but purposefully peeling back each layer of the abuse to reveal the victim's true self.

This type of systemic work will aid you in seeing the bigger picture by helping you to understand the system you were working within, the dynamics at play and your own journey thus far.

Codependency's worst characteristic is that of too much tolerance for the other and not enough for the self. You can work on how to stop blaming yourself for everything and on identifying and respecting your own needs as you move slowly along the path to healing.

Being trained by your narcissist that you are the 'problem' and you are 'wrong' will take a lot of unravelling and healing. If you have left a narcissistic spouse or romantic partner behind, be mindful that there is also a grieving process to be completed and work to be done to ensure previous patterns of relating are not repeated, either with a previous partner or someone else.

It may be that a codependent is unable to leave the relationship and decides to quit therapy instead. That is OK so long as I make it clear that I am not condoning a return to an abusive situation. When I experience this situation, I always tell the codependent that my door remains open for them. . .

RECOMMENDED READING

Brutally Honest–Melanie Brown

Desire: Where Sex Meets Addiction–Susan Cheever

Divorcing a Narcissist: Advice from the Battlefield–Tina Swithin

Escape from Intimacy–Anne Wilson Schaef

How to Do No Contact Like a Boss! The Essential Guide to Detaching from Pathological Love and Reclaiming Your Life–Kim Saeed

The Harder They Fall: Celebrities Tell Their Real-Life Stories of Addiction and Recovery–Edited by Gary Stromberg and Jane Miles

Healing Your Aloneness: Finding Love and Wholeness Through Your Inner Child–Margaret Paul and Erika J. Chopich

Guts: The Endless Follies and Tiny Triumphs of a Giant Disaster–Kristen Johnston

Splitting: Protecting Yourself While Divorcing Someone With Borderline or Narcissistic Personality Disorder–Billy Eddy and Randi Kreger

Unfiltered: No Shame, No Regrets, Just Me–Lily Collins

CHAPTER 14

A BETTER WAY TO BE: CREATING NEW BOUNDARIES TO MOVE FORWARD

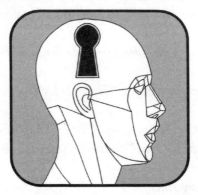

"You live the life you accept for yourself."
-Michael Padraig Acton-

Once you are physically free of a narcissist, you need to quickly create new rules for yourself, new boundaries that will protect you going forward.

How do we choose the right path? How do we avoid being led astray by another scheming parasite?

Love, unity and compassion
We must let love, unity and compassion be our guides.

We get back what we give out to the world. If we project fear and neediness, we attract and become stuck to needy, jealous and controlling narcissists. What's more, we will push most genuine and kind people away.

If we can, instead, project love out to the world, we will

attract love back to ourselves. The real love we always craved and not the sham romance of a narcissistic dance. Learn to recognise and treasure warmth and tenderness in others.

Narcissists work through isolation. Therefore, your shield is in unity with others. Strengthen your social networks and create new ones with like-minded friends. Be light-hearted and easy to be around. Respect people for their unique souls and don't focus on how they might have different views or priorities to yours. Enjoy the company of those who want to introduce you to their circle because they value your whole person—not how you look in your best outfit!

When you have come far enough along this road, you will start to understand the difference between compassion, a real empathy with another soul, and a connection based on fear and control. You will be able to give of yourself because you are overflowing, not because you need something in return.

You live the life you accept for yourself

Whenever my eye catches this quotation on my computer screen, it reminds me of a special encounter I had while living in Georgia, Atlanta over 15 years ago.

I needed a haircut and decided to jump into Supercuts. This really nice girl came over, we went through how she was going to cut my hair and then she said, "Would you mind me asking you what your favourite recipe or favourite food is?" I was quite taken aback. Through the conversation she revealed that she had a six year-old child and was on her own as a single parent. She said she loved her job and loved helping people and she just had this big glow around her.

She told me what she likes to do is ask her clients for

their recipes so that she can make something similar and take it to her church group. She collected the recipes from all these different people and there was just an aura of peace and happiness about her. It's something that really stayed with me because she is one of the most successful people I have ever met.

Why? Because she had truly accepted her life, not as a victim who was living on the breadline and had got pregnant with a man who didn't want to marry her, but as a hard-working person who gives to others. That's her success. She shares stories, she shares recipes. She joyously gives.

A narcissist only takes and the codependent gives out of fear and not joy.

My challenge to you is to refuse to accept that toxic life any more. Choose a worthier existence. Because we all truly do live the lives we accept for ourselves.

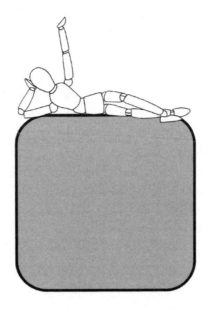

"Choose a worthier existence."
-Michael Padraig Acton-

AFTERWORD

NPD and codependency are not pretty subjects to write about. However, I hope that this book will bring relief to anyone experiencing this type of relationship. The greatest reward in doing my job is to see the relief in a person's face when they learn, understand and 'get' that they are NOT alone; NPD is a real issue and it is more common than people think.

The three major tasks in hand for a complete and lasting recovery are:

1. Understanding the true definition of dignity.
2. Healthy tolerance for self and others.
3. Serenity and healthy compassion for self and others.

Codependents, I have discovered, are missing a template on how to be with an intimate other, usually stemming from chaos when growing up or not being taught that it is OK for boundaries (regarding self and other) to exist.

After many, many years in academia and working on the front line of therapy, I've learnt so much from all the brave and engaging people I have met.

I considered joining a research team or going back into teaching. But with my family and friends scattered, and with the intensives and counselling work I do visiting people in my rooms in London and Miami, not to mention online, I felt that to restrict myself to a faculty would hinder my continuing with my chosen path: working with those who desperately want and need change.

So, after much deliberation, and working with my own

psychologist in session after session, I decided to write a series of books about common issues brought to therapy, balancing evidence-based facts about these issues with real examples of how people have worked through them to create a better life. And the *Power of You* series is born!

I have a lot of patients who have worked with me to be thankful to. If it were not for all their hard work, input and wisdom I would never have been able to write this for you and your dear ones.

Remember this: if you are thinking of leaving a narcissist then plan carefully and choose the timing to be safe and manageable.

Jackie finally left John. She couldn't lead the fake life anymore. She returned to me for more work and decided that she was an adult and made herself sustainable. She realised life could be better away from the control.

As for John, he has moved on to his next target. . .

PLEASE GIVE YOUR FEEDBACK

Thank you for reading this first book in the *Power of You* series.

- What did you like?
- What changes would you like to see?
- What topics would you like me to write about next?

I want this to continue to be the most helpful and informative book of its kind on this subject.

Please contribute by leaving a review via my contact page on my website, on Amazon, on Goodreads, and share on social media—you never know who you might help by spreading the word!

Connect with me online:
- Twitter: https://twitter.com/Actonmp
- Facebook: https://www.facebook.com/Actonmp
- Instagram: https://www.instagram.com/michael_padraig_acton/
- YouTube: https://www.youtube.com/channel/UCHGfUjqfS2ERjjKtPaQcQ5w
- LinkedIn: https://www.linkedin.com/in/michael-padraig-acton-1045562b/
- Website: https://mpamind.com
- Email: michael@mpamind.com

GLOSSARY OF TERMS

American Psychiatric Association (APA): The largest professional association of psychiatrists and trainee psychiatrists in the world. The APA publish the *Diagnostic and Statistical Manual of Mental Disorders.*

Amorous narcissist: Theodore Millon's proposed subtype of narcissist (not accepted by the APA). A narcissist who focuses their activity on the intimate relationship sphere. Seductive and sexually promiscuous.

Antisocial Personality Disorder (ASPD): A personality disorder characterised by a lack of respect for the rights of others, often involving acts of aggression and violence.

Bipolar Disorder: A disorder which causes fluctuation in mood between mania and depression.

Borderline Personality Disorder (BPD): A personality disorder characterised by extreme emotional instability and impulsive behaviour, including self-harm.

Cerebral narcissist: An unofficial narcissistic subtype where attention is manipulated largely by non-physical attributes such as intelligence and status.

Classic narcissist: An unofficial term used to contrast with proposed subtypes of narcissism.

Cluster B disorders: A grouping of personality disorders within the DSM-5, known as the 'Dramatic, emotional, erratic disorders.'

Codependency (CD): A feature of a relationship whereby one partner enables another's addiction or poor mental health.

Compensatory narcissist: Theodore Millon's proposed subtype of narcissist (not accepted by the APA). A passive narcissist who has fantasies of success and blames others for their failure.

Covert narcissist: See Compensatory Narcissist.

Domestic Abuse: A pattern of behaviour which involves one member of a domestic relationship abusing another whether physically, emotionally, sexually or in other ways.

DSM-5: The latest (2013) edition of the *Diagnostic and Statistical Manual of Mental Disorders*. Published by the APA, it standardises and classifies mental disorders.

Elitist narcissist: Theodore Millon's proposed subtype of narcissist (not accepted by the APA). A narcissist who associates with people of a privileged status without earning their place.

False ego: A false self or mask created to hide one's own insecurities.

Gaslighting: A psychological strategy used by abusers to manipulate the reality of their victims.

Grandiose Narcissist: See Classic Narcissist.

Grandiosity: An inflated sense of self-importance; one of the distinguishing features of NPD.

Histrionic Personality Disorder (HPD): A personality disorder characterised by attention-seeking behaviour, often through inappropriate sexual activity and exaggerated emotions.

Malignant Narcissist: Originally a sadistic narcissist midway along a continuum from NPD to psychopathy. Today, broadly applied to narcissists who behave antisocially.

Narcissistic Personality Disorder (NPD): A personality disorder characterised by self-obsession, an inflated sense of importance and a need for admiration.

Narcissistic rage: A display of extreme anger as a reaction to a perceived injury to a person's self-esteem.

Narcissistic supply: A source of admiration or positive attention.

Narcissus Syndrome: Where a company or organisation is destroyed by a narcissistic leader.

Obsessive compulsive disorder (OCD): An anxiety disorder characterised by repetitive behaviours.

Passive Dependent Personality (PDP): A psychoanalytic term for the personality type likely to become the victim in a narcissist-codependent relationship.

Pathology: The study of disease.

Personality disorder: A category of mental disorders characterised by maladaptive behaviours and negative inner experiences.

Psyche: The totality of the mind (conscious and unconscious); the subject of psychological study.

Sociopath: Someone who has been conditioned to behave as a psychopath by their upbringing.

Somatic narcissist: An unofficial narcissistic subtype where attention is manipulated largely by physical attributes such as sex and physical pleasure.

Symptomatology: The combined symptoms of a disease.

Syndrome: A disorder comprising a combination of different symptoms.

GLOSSARY OF TERMS continued

Trait: A quality or characteristic.

Unprincipled narcissist: Theodore Millon's proposed subtype of narcissist (not accepted by the APA). A narcissist who indulges in antisocial behaviour.

FURTHER READING

CHAPTER 1

Children of the Self-Absorbed: A Grownup's Guide to Getting Over Narcissistic Parents-Nina W. Brown

Disarming the Narcissist-Wendy Behary

Emotional Blackmail-Susan Forward

Emotional Vampires-Alan Bernstein

Malignant Self-Love: Narcissism Revisited-Sam Vaknin

The Narcissistic Family: A Guide to Diagnosis-Stephanie Pressman

Toxic Parents: Overcoming Their Hurtful Legacy and Reclaiming Your Life-Susan Forward

Trapped in the Mirror-Elan Golomb

Why Is It Always About You? The Seven Deadly Sins of Narcissism-Sandy Hotchkiss

Will I Ever Be Good Enough? Healing the Daughters of Narcissistic Mothers-Karyn McBride

CHAPTER 2

Codependents Anonymous-CODA

Codependency for Dummies-Darlene Lancer

Codependent No More-Melody Beattie

CHAPTER 3

Red Flag: 50 Warning Signs of Narcissistic Seduction-H. G. Tudor

Sitting Target: How and Why a Narcissist Chooses You-H. G. Tudor

So You're Dating a Narcissist-Sheldon Brown

When Love is a Lie: Narcissistic Partners & the Pathological Relationship Agenda-Zari Ballard

Your Brain on Love, Sex and the Narcissist: The Biochemical Bonds that Keep Us Addicted to Our Abusers-Shahida Arabi

CHAPTER 4

30 Covert Emotional Manipulation Tactics: How Manipulators Take Control in Personal Relationships-Adelyn Birch

The Covert Passive-Aggressive Narcissist-Debbie Mirza

From Charm to Harm: And Everything Else in Between With a Narcissist-Gregory Zaffuto

Gaslighting, Love Bombing and Flying Monkeys-Angela Atkinson

In Sheep's Clothing: Understanding and Dealing with Manipulative People-George Simon Jr.

Magic Words: How to Get What You Want from a Narcissist-Lindsey Ellison

Object of My Affection is in My Reflection: Coping with Narcissists-Rokelle Lerner

You Might Be a Narcissist If. . . How to Identify Narcissism in Ourselves and Others and What We Can Do About It-Cynthia Munz, Lisa Charlebois and Paul Meier

Take Control of Your Life-Daniel Jave and Frank Gerard

Codependent Cure-Jean Harrison and Beattie Grey

Stop Being Codependent in 10 Easy Steps-Catie Grandmaison

Cure Codependency and Conquer as an Empath-Leanne Walters and Carol Grace Anderson

Breaking Codependency: How to Navigate the Traps That Sabotage Your Life-Lesly Devereaux

Narcissistic Disorders in Children and Adolescents: Diagnosis and Treatment-Phyllis Beren

Raising Resilient Children with a Borderline or Narcissistic Parent-Margalis Fjelstad and Jean McBride

Narcissistic Parents: Why Emotionally Immature Parents Infantilise Their Children-Cecilia Overt

Children and Narcissistic Personality Disorder: A Guide for Parents-Cynthia Bailey-Rug

Co-Parenting with a Toxic Ex-Amy J.L. Baker ph.D, Raul R. Fine LCSW, et al.

Dealing with Emotionally Immature Parents: How to Handle Toxic Parents-Priscilla Posey and Robin Howatt Shrock

Narcissistic Mothers-Elizabeth Ex

The Narcissistic Family: Diagnosis and Treatment-Stephanie Donaldson-Pressman and Robert M. Pressman

Narcissistic Mothers-Michelle Evans, Angela Peel, et al.

Education in a Narcissistic Nation: Build Foundations for Students, Not Pedestals-Karen Brackman and Chad Mason

CHAPTER 9

Do you Work for a Narcissistic Organization? https://www.psychologytoday.com/us/blog/your-personal-renaissance/201804/do-you-work-narcissistic-organization

How to Work for a Narcissistic Boss https://hbr.org/2016/04/how-to-work-for-a-narcissistic-boss

Narcissistic Leaders: The Incredible Pros, the Inevitable Cons https://hbr.org/2004/01/narcissistic-leaders-the-incredible-pros-the-inevitable-cons

How Does Leader Narcissism Influence Employee Voice: The Attribution of Leader Impression Management and Leader-Member Exchange https://www.ncbi.nlm.nih.gov/pmc/articles/PMC6571719/

Narcissistic Leadership: How to Identify Narcissists and Cope with Narcissism at Work https://www.ckju.net/en/blog/narcissistic-leadership-how-identify-narcissists-and-cope-narcissism-work/31265

Detaching Yourself from a Codependent Relationship https://www.kanecountydivorceattorneys.com/st-charles-lawyers/codependent-relationship

CHAPTER 12

Break Free: Disarm, Defeat, and Beat The Narcissist and Psychopath–Pamela Kole

Escape: How to Beat the Narcissist–H. G. Tudor

Exorcism: Purging the Narcissist from Heart and Soul–H. G. Tudor

Healing from Hidden Abuse: A Journey Through the Stages of Recovery from Psychological Abuse-Shannon Thomas

Healing from a Narcissistic Relationship: A Caretaker's Guide to Recovery, Empowerment, and Transformation-Margalis Fjelstad

The Journey: A Roadmap for Self-Healing After Narcissistic Abuse-Meredith Miller

No Contact With the Narcissist: Escaping Narcissism & Narcissistic Personality Disorder-James Aniston

Run Sis: A Survivor's Guide for Escaping Narcissistic Abuse-Charisma Deberry

Revenge: How to Beat the Narcissist-H. G. Tudor

Whole Again: Healing Your Heart and Rediscovering Your True Self After Toxic Relationships and Emotional Abuse-Jackson MacKenzie

CHAPTER 13

Brutally Honest-Melanie Brown

Desire: Where Sex Meets Addiction-Susan Cheever

Divorcing a Narcissist: Advice from the Battlefield-Tina Swithin

Escape from Intimacy-Anne Wilson Schaef

How to Do No Contact Like a Boss! The Essential Guide to Detaching from Pathological Love and Reclaiming Your Life-Kim Saeed

The Harder They Fall: Celebrities Tell Their Real-Life Stories of Addiction and Recovery-Edited by Gary Stromberg and Jane Miles

Healing Your Aloneness: Finding Love and Wholeness Through Your Inner Child-Margaret Paul and Erika J. Chopich

Guts: The Endless Follies and Tiny Triumphs of a Giant Disaster-Kristen Johnston

Splitting: Protecting Yourself While Divorcing Someone With Borderline or Narcissistic Personality Disorder-Billy Eddy and Randi Kreger

Unfiltered: No Shame, No Regrets, Just Me-Lily Collins

ENDNOTES

1. Personality Disorders factsheet, www.dsm5.org, published 2013, last accessed 17/11/2014

2 *The Dark Triad of Personality: Narcissism, Machiavellianism, and Psychopathy*, Journal of Research in Personality, Academic Press, published 2002

ABOUT MICHAEL PADRAIG ACTON

Michael Padraig Acton (B.Ed., M.Ed. (Psych.) Hons., M.A. C.Psych., P.D. C.Psych., BPSsS., BACP (Accred), MICF) is a consultant, psychological therapist, counsellor, clinical supervisor, legal consultant, systemic life coach, trained scientist practitioner and author with over 30 years of clinical experience. Working globally, with his main offices in London (UK) and Fort Lauderdale (US), originally from England and Ireland, Michael specialises in helping couples, families and individuals. He has extensive training in approaches including applied clinical and counselling psychology, CBT, psychoanalysis and psychodynamic, Jungian, Gestalt, systemic and transactional analysis, as well as holistic forms of therapeutic alliance such as mindfulness and shamanism.

As mostly a single parent for his daughter's upbringing and having no parental support as a child, Michael left home and the Catholic church behind at the age of 17 having spent months struggling to survive meningitis. Despite being homeless and sleeping rough in a friend's car, Michael had a moment of realisation that for the first time in his life he was completely free. He moved into a tiny bedsit with a shared kitchen and bathroom in Gravesend, Kent, working as a waiter and barman to make ends meet, before deciding to pursue a career as a teacher. This took him around the world.

After experiencing counselling psychology in Australia, both as a client and a pastoral care provider at the college where he taught, he soon realised his future lay in that direction. He applied for a conversion course to become a graduate member of the British Psychological Society and went through clinical training at Dundee University.

Michael's first clinical role was at Dundee Royal Infirmary, before moving to Sussex to study, work and research alongside Dr Mick Burton and Professor Mic Cooper on psychodynamic and family/young person's therapy. Michael has worked within the NHS in pain management and drug dependency units, adolescent and young people's clinics and with Relate's couples counselling programmes, in addition to counselling HIV and AIDS patients for a charity.

In 1998, Michael was asked by The London Institute to set up a private practice in West London based upon his work experience with families, couples and substance abuse; identity issues; life crises, and gender dysphoria, as well as his research and work with lesbian, gay and bisexual issues. In 2004, he took a sabbatical to work and travel in America and Australia. During this time he researched suicide prevalence and prevention and worked with shamanism alongside native people. After his sabbatical, he returned to the UK to resume his practice, and be close to his daughter and grandchildren. He now continues to divide his time between the UK and the USA. Michael still travels worldwide to support people in his consultant's role. All his work is enveloped by Rogerian core values of empowerment and the importance of the therapeutic integrative relationship. Michael is a genuine, caring and thoughtful professional, dad and grandpa with scholastic and real human values.

For more information: www.MPAmind.com.